Spinal Injuries Handbook

Hugh Dickson MB BS, FACRM
Director of Rehabilitation, Liverpool Hospital,
New South Wales

David Martens BSocStud
Social Worker, Spinal Injuries Unit,
The Prince Henry Hospital,
New South Wales

Louise Dever BSW
Social Worker, Commonwealth Rehabilitation Services,
New South Wales
formerly Social Worker, The Prince Henry Hospital,
New South Wales

Jann Tonkin BSW
formerly Spinal Injuries Worker,
The Prince Henry Hospital, New South Wales

McGRAW-HILL BOOK COMPANY Sydney
New York San Francisco Auckland Bogotá
Caracas Lisbon London Madrid Mexico City
Milan Montreal New Delhi San Juan
Singapore Tokyo Toronto

Text, design and format copyright © 1993 McGraw-Hill Book Company Australia Pty Limited
Illustrations copyright © CIBA-GEIGY 1987

**National Library of Australia
Cataloguing-in-Publication data:**

The Prince Henry Hospital spinal injuries handbook.

    3rd ed.
    Includes index.
    ISBN 0 07 470001 4.

    1. Spinal cord—Wounds and injuries—Patients—Rehabilitation—New South Wales. 2. Spine—Wounds and injuries—Patients—Rehabilitation—New South Wales. I. Dickson, Hugh. II. Prince Henry Hospital (Little Bay, NSW). III. Title. Spinal injuries handbook.

362.43809944

Produced in Australia by McGraw-Hill Book Company Australia Pty Limited, 4 Barcoo Street, Roseville, NSW 2069, Australia
Printed in Australia by Globe Press Pty Ltd, Victoria
Sponsoring Editor: Nichola Dyson
Production Editor: Avril Janks
Designer: George Sirett

Foreword

Hi,

My name is David Guest. Up until two years ago when a simple motorcycle ride to the local shopping centre went wrong, I was leading the life of your average single twenty-seven-year-old.

I was a self-employed electrical contractor working long hours so I could play long hours.

That afternoon I was torn out of that world and thrown into a world that most people couldn't conceive.

For the next six and a half months my home became the Spinal Injuries Unit at Prince Henry Hospital.

Sustaining a spinal injury, in my case C4 quadriplegia, has meant forgetting everything about life that came naturally and starting from scratch. Before my accident I didn't even know what a quadriplegic or paraplegic was, nor did my family and friends. Yet when I became a quadriplegic we were all expected to learn about this new world in a very short space of time.

The *Spinal Injuries Handbook* was for me the book with all the answers. It supplemented and reinforced the enormous amount of information that I was expected to absorb.

For my family and friends it was the main source of information about my injury—what it meant and what the future would hold. Also, it gave all of us concrete information about the support services I would be using and the direction I would be heading in my rehabilitation.

Now two years down the track I am living out in the community by myself, as independently as possible. I've completed a number of TAFE courses and am

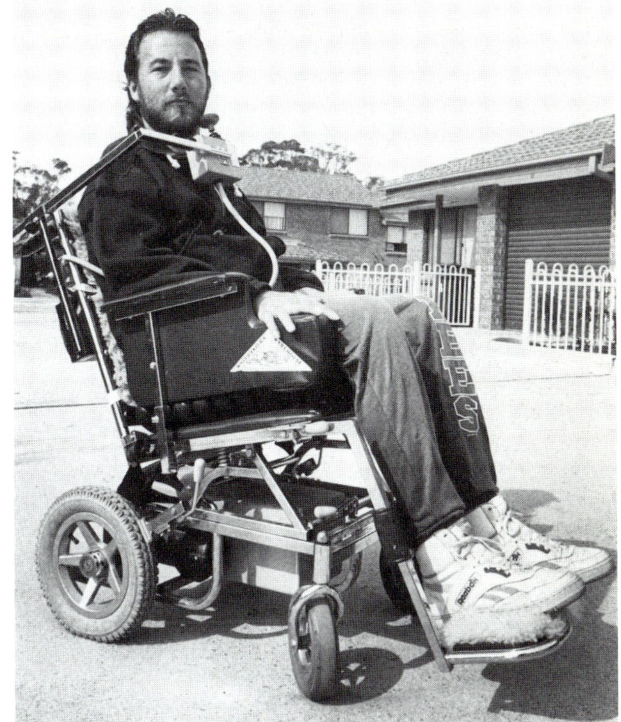

currently studying advanced computer-aided drafting with the aim of regaining, sometime in the near future, self-employment in this new field.

I know this book will be a valuable tool for those people both directly and indirectly affected by spinal injury.

DAVID GUEST

Contents

8 Rehabilitation and work

9 Accommodation

10 Finances

11 Compensation for personal injury

12 Equipment

13 Support associations

14 Transportation

15 Recreation

16 Discrimination—knowing your rights

Acknowledgments

We wish to thank the following for their contribution to this edition of the *Prince Henry Hospital Spinal Injuries Handbook:*

Richard Jones, Director, Spinal Injuries Unit, Prince Henry Hospital, Sydney

Michelle Pokorra, Pharmacist, Prince Henry Hospital, Sydney

Liliana Calabrese, formerly Social Worker, Spinal Injuries Unit, Prince Henry Hospital, Sydney

Julie Wilson, Occupational Therapist

Christine O'Hara, Social Worker, Royal Perth Rehabilitation Hospital

Peter Trethewey, Social Worker, Austin Hospital, Victoria

Pat Dorsett, Social Worker, Princess Alexandra Hospital, Queensland

Sue Hansen, Social Worker, Spinal Unit, Royal Adelaide Hospital, South Australia

Karen Gosling, Social Worker, Spinal Rehabilitation Unit, Hampstead Centre, South Australia

Motor Accidents Authority of New South Wales
Law Society of New South Wales

We would also like to thank the following organisations for permission to use information from their brochures and booklets:

Legal Aid Commission of New South Wales
Sporting Injuries Committee (New South Wales)
WorkCover Authority of New South Wales

(Note to the reader: The information supplied by WorkCover is a general guide to workers' compensation and related matters in New South Wales, and does not claim to be exhaustive. Legislation changes regularly, and you should consult your legal advisor in relation to specific rights or responsibilities.)

Anti-Discrimination Board of New South Wales (Information supplied is correct as of June, 1991.)

Victims Compensation Tribunal of New South Wales (The information on the Victims Compensation Scheme in Chapter 11, pp. 64–6, is derived from the pamphlet 'Compensation to Victims of Violent Crime' (Crown copyright), and reproduced with the permission of the Crown.)

We would especially like to thank the Social Work Department at Prince Henry Hospital, Sydney, for their support, and in particular we would like to thank Ms Cynthia Mansell and Mrs Anne Haines for their assistance in typing and preparing the manuscript.

Introduction to the third edition

Five years have elapsed since I wrote an Introduction to the first edition of *The Prince Henry Hospital Spinal Injuries Handbook*. At that time I eulogised the efforts of Sir Ludwig Guttman and emphasised the importance of specialised spinal units for providing comprehensive care to paraplegics and quadriplegics. Much has been achieved to normalise the lives of men and women suffering the permanent effects of spinal cord injury, and the *Handbook* set out information on the anatomical aspects of spinal cord injury and our current knowledge about the management of bladder and bowel and sexual impairment. The first edition also discussed equipment for improving the quality of life and independence in personal care and the activities of daily living. It listed contacts for ongoing community involvement and social, recreational and vocational pursuits.

I emphasised that much remained to be done in the community to improve opportunities for the spinal injured and their access to services. Since then there has been enormous progress, but I must emphasise that the achievements of our community are not etched in granite; these achievements are vulnerable to attack, to erosion, and, indeed, to reversal. It is necessary to emphasise the risks inherent in our complacency and to encourage all of us to maintain our enthusiasm and our lobbying in order to ensure that what we have already achieved is retained and that further independence in the community is guaranteed. Persons with spinal cord damage can then be given their rightful opportunity to participate and to achieve their ambitions, gaining the greatest achievements of which they are capable.

We have many challenges for the future, and it is important that plans be laid now for facilities for people with spinal cord injury. In this way they will have the care that is required as they feel the effects of the ageing process—these occur to them at a faster rate than we might expect for their chronological age. While I believe that it is possible to participate actively well into old age, there will undoubtedly be increasing disability, and we must emphasise the need to plan now for the future. A greater number of high-level quadriplegics are surviving their injuries and requiring support with high-technology equipment. Accommodation options must be varied and must range from hostel to family accommodation; it will, in general, best be provided by voluntary organisations.

While attendant care has been a worthwhile initiative, the program has stalled, perhaps due to economic stringencies. However, I believe that the eligibility of the present scheme should be broadened and, if the program is seen to be successful, greater funding should be provided.

There remains in persons with spinal cord injury considerable, untapped energy for vocational activities. Therefore, both the workplace and transportation systems need to be made more accessible to people with impairments. Unless there is greater flexibility with disability allowances and income derived from vocational endeavours, there will always be a disincentive to open employment. The cost of items required recurrently, including medications and aids, is high, and is further affected by loss of eligibility for financial assistance when people return to work after severe injuries. The PADP scheme has failed to live up to the expectations created by its promotion in 1981, the International Year of the Disabled.

There have been remarkable improvements in the prevention of injuries in motor vehicles, with the improved design of lap-sash safety belts, and there is now legislation to provide lap-sash integrated seat belts in tourist coaches. The rules of rugby have been progressively modified, and our community is more aware of the dangers of diving into shallow pools, of high-speed water sports, and the effects of alcohol and drugs. There is, however, much to be done in the area of substance abuse and its effects on people both on the roads and involved in sporting activities.

There have been major advances in the medical management of spinal cord injuries, including implantable pumps for the administration of medications to control spasticity and pain, the electrical control of bladder emptying, the functional electrical stimulation of peripheral nerves and the nerves supplying the diaphragm to improve muscle performance, and improvements in fertility management, with programs for the collection of sperm of apparently infertile male spinal-injured persons. Also, space technology has reached into the areas of appliances and environmental control systems.

Many of these achievements have been procured through the initiatives of the Paraplegic and Quadriplegic Association of New South Wales and the Australian Quadriplegic Association, and the many voluntary organisations that are dedicated to improving the lifestyle of people with impairments.

Let us work together toward further improvements and prevent any retraction of rights already gained. This will improve not only the quality of life of the spinal injured, but also the lifestyle of those who are not physically impaired.

ASSOCIATE PROFESSOR RICHARD F. JONES
Director, Spinal Injury Unit
The Prince Henry Hospital
Sydney, Australia

CHAPTER 1

Spinal cord injury

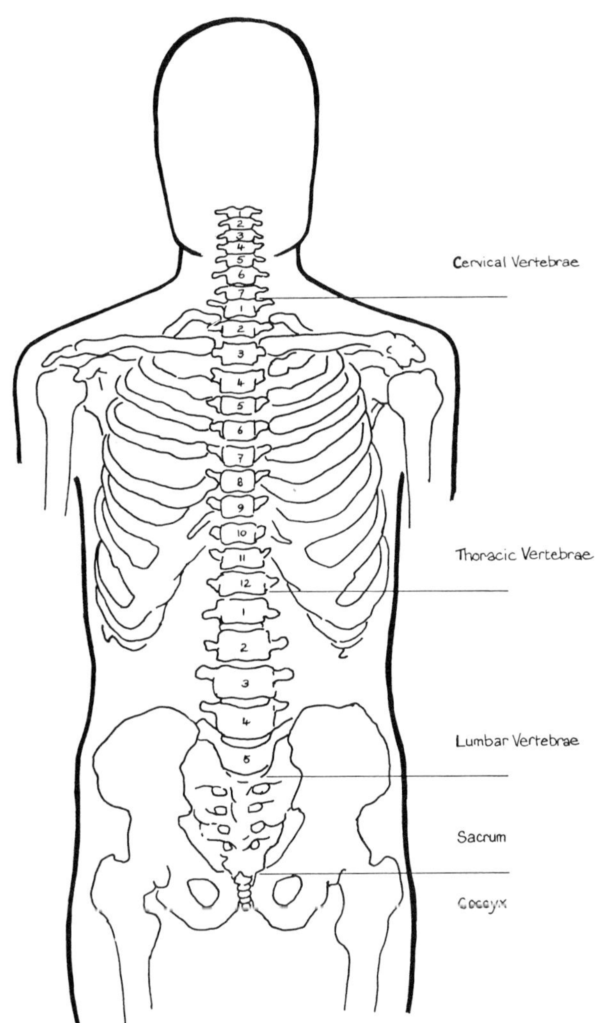

Fig. 1.1 The spine: vertebral column

What is the spine?

The spine is a series of bones that run from the pelvis to the skull, carrying the load of the body and the head.

The bones of the neck are called the **cervical vertebrae**, the bones of the upper back that are in line with the chest are called the **thoracic vertebrae** and the bones of the lower back are called the **lumbar vertebrae**. Parts of each vertebra rest on the vertebrae above and below it. These parts are the **joints,** and they keep the vertebrae in their correct position and in alignment with each other. Each vertebra is separated from the next vertebra by a spinal shock absorber called a **disc**. In the canal running in the rear of the vertebrae is the **spinal cord**.

■ The spinal cord

The spinal cord is part of the nervous system. It contains thousands and thousands of microscopic, delicate nerve cells, and long extensions of the cells called nerve fibres.

The structure of the cord is very complex. Brain cells connect to cells in the cord, which are then connected by their fibres to muscles and to various sensory receptors. The system operates continuously to regulate the activities of the body. Some of the processing of information and control of activity is done by the brain, and some by centres in the cord. Most of this goes on without the person being aware of it. It is not necessary, for instance, to have to think about digesting a meal or which finger to move next when scratching.

The nerve cells and their fibres need food and oxygen to keep them working. This is brought to them by blood vessels.

The spinal cord floats in a fluid called cerebro-spinal fluid. It is protected by this means from bumping the wall of the spinal canal, as it has its weight supported by flotation. The whole structure is supported as well by a series of protective membranes.

The cord can be divided into segments from the top down, corresponding to the point of exit and entry of the major bundles of nerve fibres. These bundles are called nerve roots.

After leaving the cord, the nerve roots combine with each other to form the peripheral nerves. The nerves run to the muscles and other structures, conveying impulses (electro-chemical signals) to and from the cord and brain. Each segment of the cord supplies a set group of muscles, joints, skin area and internal organs. The functions and importance of the different segments will be seen in the section on spinal injury.

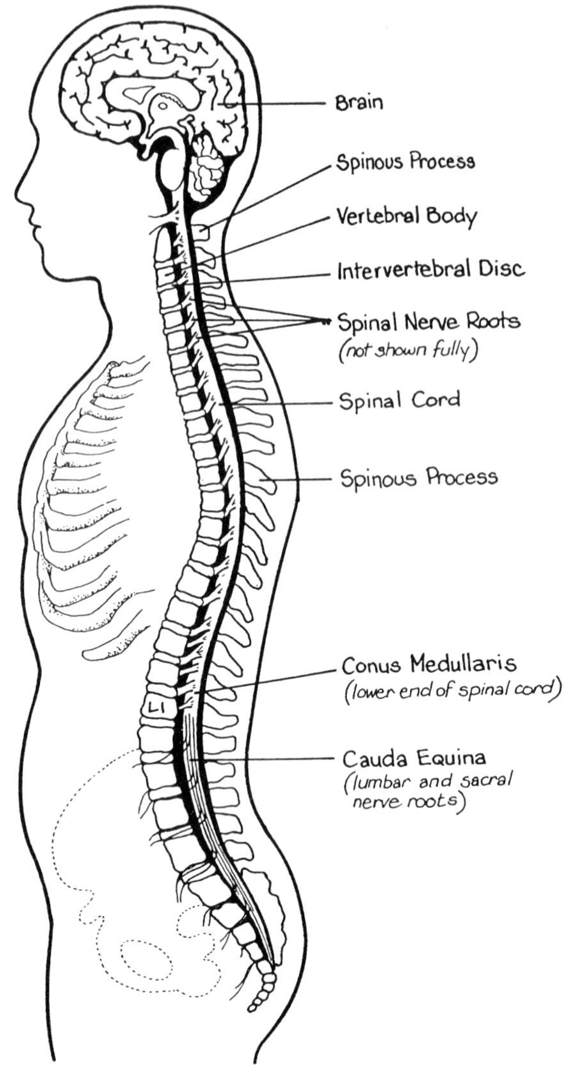

Fig. 1.2 The spinal cord

Spinal injury

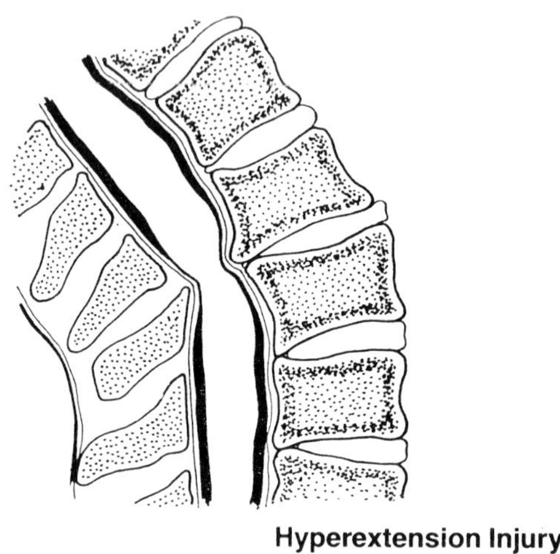

A spinal injury may result in:

1. injury to bones and the joints between them, and/or
2. injury to the spinal cord, either by a direct blow that crushes the delicate fibres, or by damage to the blood vessels. Damage means that the microscopic cells of food and oxygen have been starved and killed.

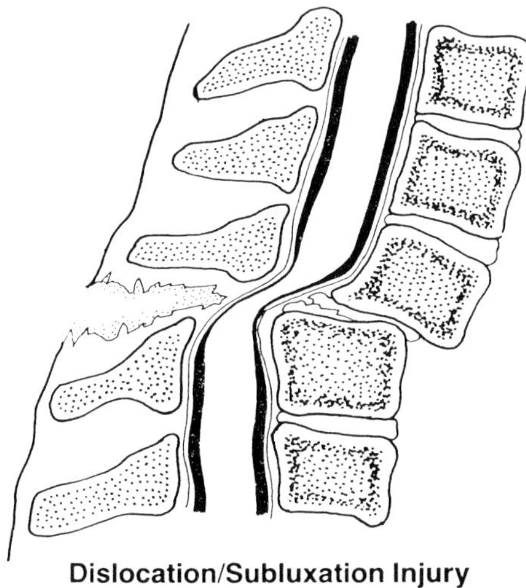

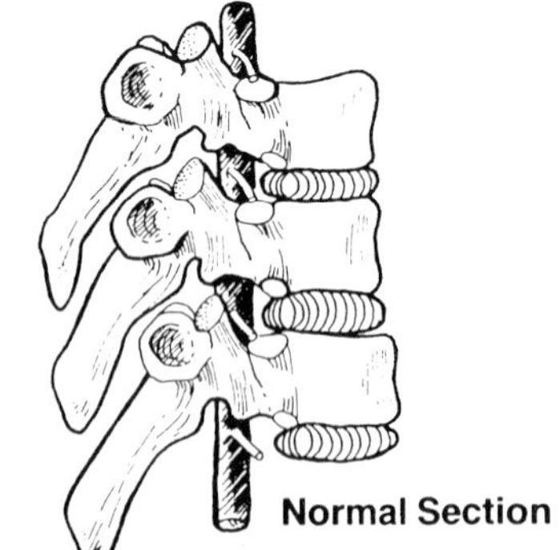

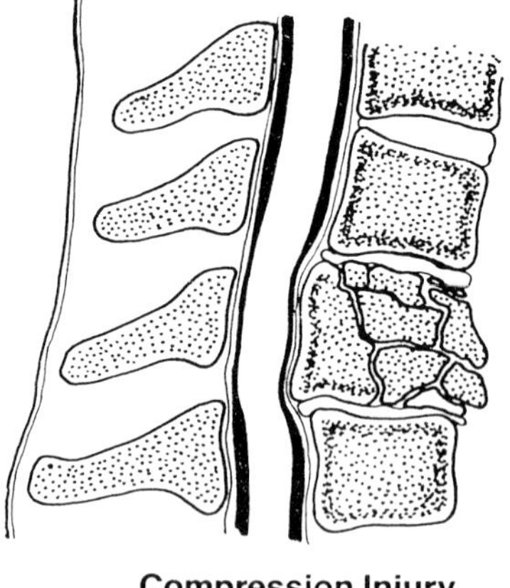

Fig. 1.3 (a) to (d) Injuries to the spinal cord

It is possible to injure the bones without injury to the spinal cord, and vice versa. Children and old people, especially, can injure their cord without injury to their bones.

■ Injury to the vertebrae

The main problem in an injury to the vertebrae is usually the damage to the joints rather than to the bones. If a joint is damaged so that it has been moved from its normal position, this is called a dislocation. An incomplete dislocation is called a subluxation. In these situations, pulling on the joints will realign them. This pulling process is called **traction.**

Breaks in bones are called fractures. Fractures are treated by realigning bones, by traction if necessary. When the bones are in the right place again, the fracture (or dislocation) is said to be reduced.

Sometimes an operation is necessary to bring the bones back into the right alignment.

After the bones and joints have been realigned, the realigned position must be maintained while healing takes place. This is usually done by a combination of rest in bed, perhaps traction during this time, and then the wearing of a collar or brace.

Bed rest usually lasts from six to eight weeks, depending on the patient's circumstances. The ligaments that help to hold the joints together may be torn by the injury. Often ligaments do not heal well. They are particularly prone to stretching, and after apparently healing well may allow the bones to move excessively.

This excessive movement may damage the cord, and is called instability. The stability of the fractures and joints is shown by moving the area while watching it on an x-ray screen. Frequent x-rays are taken after an injury to watch for signs of instability. If instability is detected then an operation to stop the joint from moving may be necessary. This operative procedure is called fusion.

If the area is stable, the patient is allowed up, wearing a collar or brace. This is worn for six to eight weeks, again depending on the individual's circumstances. With fractures of the lower back, however, a brace may be necessary for many months.

■ Spinal cord injury

The spinal cord may be bruised by a bone fragment, the blood supply to the cord may be damaged or the cord may be completely crushed or even severed. The degree to which the functions of the cord are lost will depend on the severity of the damage. The degree of damage will immediately be obvious as a disturbance in the ability to move the limbs or as a disturbance in sensation, or both. In a severe injury, all movements below the site of damage may be lost, as well as all sensations.

Complete injury

In a complete injury, there is loss of all movement and sensation below the level of the spinal cord injury.

Incomplete injury

An incomplete injury means that some of the pathways through the level of injury have been spared. There may be some sensation below the level of injury, or some movement of the muscles.

Spinal shock

Immediately after complete injuries and severe incomplete injuries, the cells below the level of injury will temporarily stop working, so reflex activity in that part of the cord will also be temporarily stopped. Activities in the body that depend on that reflex activity will cease until the cells in the cord that are not damaged start working again.

The process of cells 'turning off' temporarily below the level of the injury is called 'spinal shock'. The time this lasts varies from person to person. In some people, it may be only a few hours, and in others several weeks. In spinal shock, the stomach, for instance, will stop working, and any attempt to eat will result in vomiting.

Level of injury

The level of spinal cord injury is named by the last normal spinal cord segment. For injury at the T5 level, all spinal cord functions are intact down to the fifth thoracic segment. At C7, all levels are intact down to and including C7, and so on.

Quadriplegia

A quadriplegic has his or her injury at the level of the neck or cervical cord segments. Quadriplegia means paralysis or weakness in all four limbs.

Paraplegia

A paraplegic has a level of injury *below* the cervical cord segments. Paraplegia means paralysis or weakness in the *legs.*

Paraplegia or quadriplegia may be complete or incomplete. If movements are only weakened, the terms paraparesis and quadriparesis are sometimes used.

■ Cauda equina injury

The spinal cord stops at the lower border of the first lumbar vertebra. The lumbar and sacral nerve roots then run in the spinal canal from the cord down to their exit points. Anatomists fancifully considered that the bundle of nerve roots looked like a horse's tail, so they named it that in Latin—*cauda equina.*

Cauda equina injuries are injuries of the nerve roots, not of the cord. These nerve roots are connected to the muscles of the legs and pelvic region. In injuries of the lower back, the nerve roots may be damaged as they run within the spinal canal in this part of the spine.

The nerve roots are more hardy than the spinal cord, and may recover function if repaired, or if compression from bone or disc is removed. Sometimes, of course, the damage is too severe for significant recovery to take place.

Recovery

There is no such thing as a 'good' spinal injury. None of us in our right minds would want to break our necks or backs.

Of course, there are degrees of severity of spinal injury. But this is not the only factor affecting recovery. The long-term effects on lifestyle are as dependent on the mental make-up of the individual as they are on the severity of the injury.

■ Factors affecting recovery

1. The damage to the cord is immediately obvious as disturbance of function. The impairment of sensation and movement of body parts is determined by the area of spinal cord that has been damaged.

2. Healing in spinal cord lesions is usually most rapid in the first three months after injury.

3. The greater the damage to the cord, the less chance there is of recovery.

4. If all sensation and movement below the level of the injury have been lost, the chances for full recovery are very small.

5. The longer the period of no recovery, the less likely recovery is.

6. The slower the recovery, the more likely it is that recovery will be incomplete.

7. Minor changes may occur up to two years after an injury.

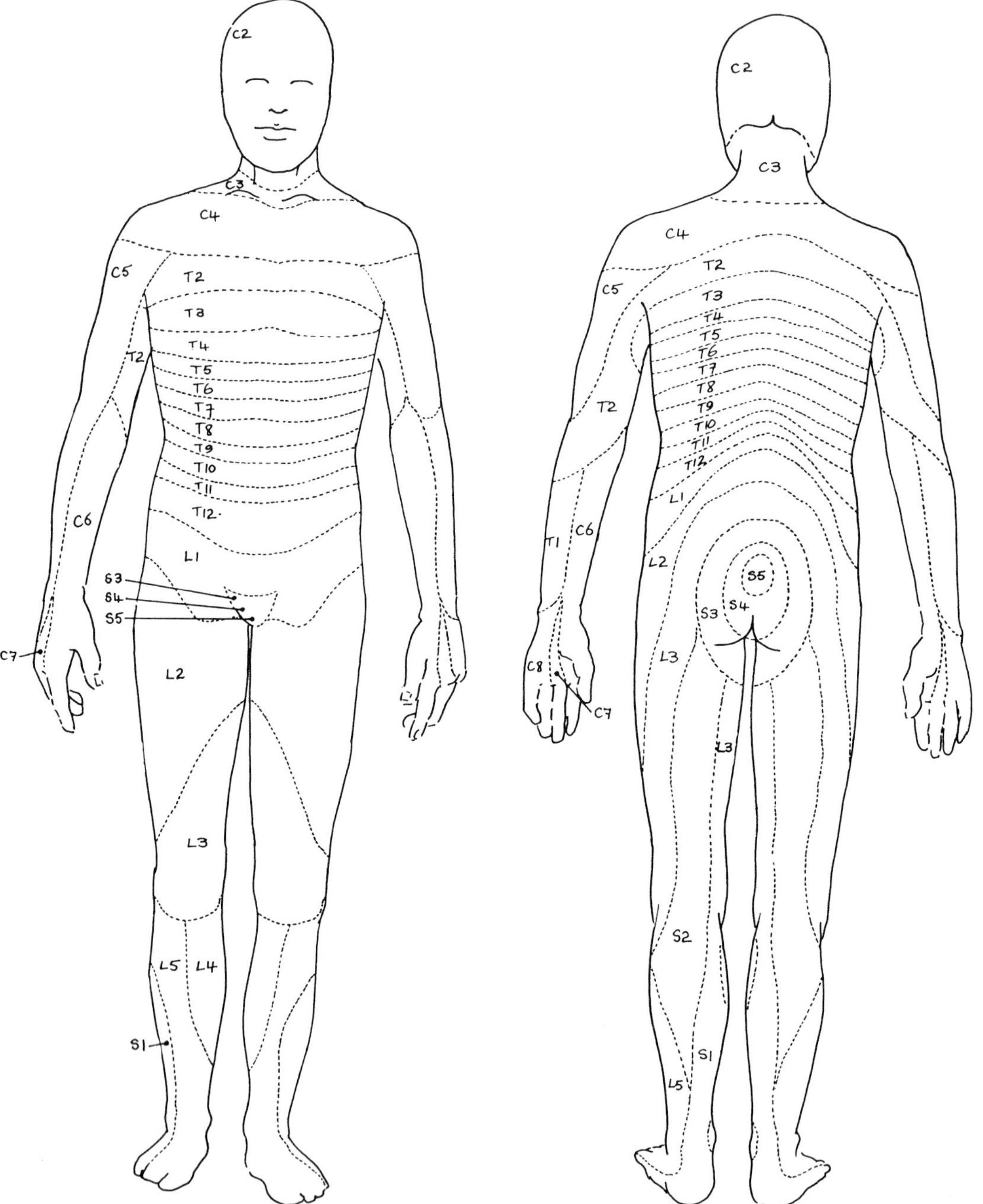

Fig. 1.4 Sensory levels

CHAPTER 2

How does a spinal cord injury affect your body?

Many activities in the body depend largely on control from the spinal cord, with messages from the brain modifying or controlling the spinal systems. If impulses from the brain cannot reach their targets in the spinal cord, the system will no longer be under full control and may be either overactive or underactive. Sensation, movement, sexual function, the bladder, bowels, heart, lungs and control of temperature may be affected.

Expected levels of function

Prior to a spinal cord injury we take our independence with many tasks for granted. We dress ourselves, feed ourselves, shave ourselves, do our hair and apply make-up. In the area of personal hygiene, we shower, clean our teeth and care for our bladders and bowels with little thought about what we are doing. Driving, moving from one place to another, carrying out household duties and communicating are all performed as part of our normal routine.

Following a spinal cord injury, our ability to perform these tasks will depend on the level of injury and on the extent to which the spinal cord is damaged. Given a particular level of injury, it is possible to predict with a fair degree of accuracy the degree of independence that can be achieved.

It is possible, then, to suggest, for those who have had complete lesions (i.e. complete injuries to the spinal cord), the levels of possible achievement in relation to their levels of injury. However, many factors affect achievement of these goals, including:

- length of time since injury
- degree of spasticity (the extent to which muscles spasm involuntarily)
- tolerance for physical strengthening
- age
- presence of other, associated injuries (e.g. fractures, head injuries)
- body build and, to some degree, pre-existing personality, self-drive and motivation
- support from family and friends
- financial status

With incomplete lesions, it is more difficult to make predictions as to an individual's level of function, because of the complex pattern or way in which sensation and movement may return over time.

As a general principle, it can be said that the lower the level of the lesions, the greater the function (see Table 2.1: Level of lesion and independence level on page 6).

Sensation

There are several kinds of sensation, such as pain, temperature, the sense of where your joints are in space—*'proprioception'*—and touch—*'light'* and *'deep'*. (Light touch means being able to feel something against your skin, such as a cotton ball or a sleeve, while deep touch means being able to feel something heavier, such as a heavy book resting on the leg.) Some structures in the body, such as the bowel, heart and bladder, have part of their nerve supplies running outside the spinal cord. Different sensations travel up different pathways in the cord. Therefore, depending on the exact site of the injury within the spinal cord, some sensations may be spared while others are damaged.

Loss of sensation or alteration in sensation is a very serious disturbance to the body. Sensations trigger reflexes that move the body when the environment is unpleasant. If sensation is lost (or the reflexes lost), damage to the skin, for example, can easily occur from burns, sharp objects or prolonged pressure.

Skin care

People with spinal injuries need to take particularly good care of their skin, so that it remains unbroken and healthy.

■ Why is healthy skin important?

Unless the skin is cared for properly, pressure areas will develop. When this happens the skin may die at the point of pressure, and ulcers will form.

Table 2.1 *Level of lesion and independence level*

Level of lesion	Movement	Level of independence
C1–3	Head and neck only (few survive, as there are respiratory complications	**Self-care:** Totally dependent **Mobility:** Chin-controlled electric wheelchair **Other equipment:** Respiratory apparatus, Environmental Control Unit
C4	Movement of head and neck and some movement of shoulders	**Self-care:** Mobile arm supports used to hold arms up against gravity and splints used to keep wrists stable. Some people are able to feed themselves, drink from adapted cups, clean their teeth and shave when set up with adapted cutlery, toothbrush and shaver. These activities are very difficult **Other activities:** Able to type using mouthstick and typewriter **Mobility:** Chin-controlled electric wheelchair on flat ground, and on ramps of low gradient **Other equipment:** Environment Control Unit to operate appliances. Can use specialist telephones
C5	Movement of head and neck. Good shoulder control. Some movement in elbow and forearm	**Self care:** With use of splints able to feed self, drink from adapted cup, clean teeth and shave when set up with adapted cutlery, toothbrush and shaver. Able to do hair with adapted extended comb. Dressing top half of body is possible **Other activities:** Typing with typing splints or sticks. Writing with splint. Rarely able to drive a car **Mobility:** Manual wheelchair very difficult, capstan knobs on handrims used. Hand-operated wheelchair usually preferred
C6	Head and neck movement. Good shoulder control. Some movement in wrist. During an extended period following the injury, the individual is usually able to develop some type of grip (although fairly weak) simply by using the natural movement of the wrist, bringing the fingers together. After a period during which the finger tendons shorten a little, allowing them to remain bent, utensils may be 'threaded' through the fingers, avoiding the need for a palmar band (though that will usually be necessary during the time in hospital	**Self-care:** Using a palmar band, able to feed self and clean teeth. Able to use adapted cup for drinking, and shaving mit for razor. Can dress top half of body, and lower half with minimal assistance. Can transfer independently from wheelchair to bed and bed to commode, but usually needs minimal assistance with other transfers **Other activities:** Able to drive car using hand controls and type, write and use the telephone—initially with aids. Domestic duties: at the least, basic tasks possible **Mobility:** Independent, using manual wheelchair with capstan knobs on handrims (occasionally may choose to use an electric wheelchair, hand-controlled for long-distance travel)
C7	Head and neck movement. Good shoulder control. Full elbow movement. Full wrist movement. Movement at fingers	**Self-care:** Should be independent in all activities: dressing, feeding, cleaning teeth, shaving and transferring on/off bed, commode (from wheelchair) and toilet, and in/out of car **Other activities:** Able to drive car using hand controls. Able to type, write, and use telephone without aids **Mobility:** Independent, using manual wheelchair. Also able to mount curbs
C8–T1	Head and neck movement. Good shoulder control. Full elbow movement. Full wrist movement. Movement in fingers. Movement in thumbs	Totally independent in all activities
T2–T12	Normal movement of upper limbs. Effect on balance depends on the level—the higher the level the worse the balance because of loss of trunk muscle control	Totally independent in all activities. May be able to stand and walk with extensive lower-limb bracing and crutches. Energy cost for walking is very high (rapidly exhausted). Can drive a car with hand controls

Table 2.1 *Level of lesion and independence level (continued)*

Level of lesion	Movement	Level of independence
T12	Paralysis of lower limbs, but good trunk control and normal upper-limb control	Energy cost for walking with braces and crutches is reasonable. Can climb stairs
L1–L3	Flexion of hip, improving as injury level descends. Knee extension improves as level descends	Walking easier, but extensive leg bracing and crutches still required

Damage to tissue deep within the skin can occur without the skin itself breaking down. A cavity may form under the skin where deep tissue has died. This cavity is called a **bursa.**

Healing a large pressure area requires a long period of rest, with no pressure on the affected area. This usually means rest in bed at home or hospital, which will interfere with independence and a normal lifestyle.

■ How is skin care achieved?

This is done by:
- prevention of pressure
- cleanliness
- keeping the skin dry, for example after showers
- protection from damage, for example from bumping the feet or sustaining injuries during transfer
- regular inspection of your skin

■ What is a pressure sore?

A pressure sore is any tissue damage caused by pressure. As we have already said, tissue damage may occur without the skin being broken. Red areas on the skin that do not fade within a few minutes are areas of tissue damage.

Forces and friction as skin is pulled over a surface are thought to increase the effect of pressure as a cause of sores. Care in sliding over sheets or on and off chairs is necessary to reduce these forces.

Development of a pressure area or sore

This is how a pressure sore develops:
- **Pressure:** pressure closes blood vessels, just as standing on a hose cuts off the water supply through it. Having no blood flowing in them for too long will damage tissues.
- **Red area:** reduced circulation in the skin leads to red areas. The redness is due to increased blood flow to the area as a response to tissue damage. The first tissue to be damaged in pressure sores is the tissue under the skin. The skin

itself is usually the last to die.
- **Open sore:** if pressure continues, then the skin begins to die. This will be shown by an ulcer developing.

Test for pressure areas

If you see a red area has developed, touch it. If the area turns white easily, this means the blood supply is still good and the tissue will heal rapidly. If it stays red, this means tissue damage has occurred and the damage will take longer to heal.

Remember:
- Most pressure sores are preventable.
- Where there is no pressure there will be no sore.
- Regular turns while in bed (every two hours) and lifts (every 15 minutes) when up in a chair are essential. You must be aware of this, and if you are unable to lift yourself or cannot be lifted by someone you know, ask someone else, even if you have to explain what to do.
- Constant checking of your skin is important to detect pressure areas early. You must either do this yourself or remind your family to do so.
- Sheepskins, boots, cushions, special beds and special mattresses may all be used to prevent sores.

Why am I prone to pressure areas?

These may be the reasons:
- poor circulation, which leads to a reduced oxygen supply to the skin
- loss of body weight (muscle and fat), which leads to the loss of protective padding over bony prominences
- inadequate pressure care, that is, not lifting or being lifted enough

Areas prone to pressure

As Figure 2.2 indicates, these areas are:
- the shoulder blades
- the elbows

(a) Normal Skin Layers

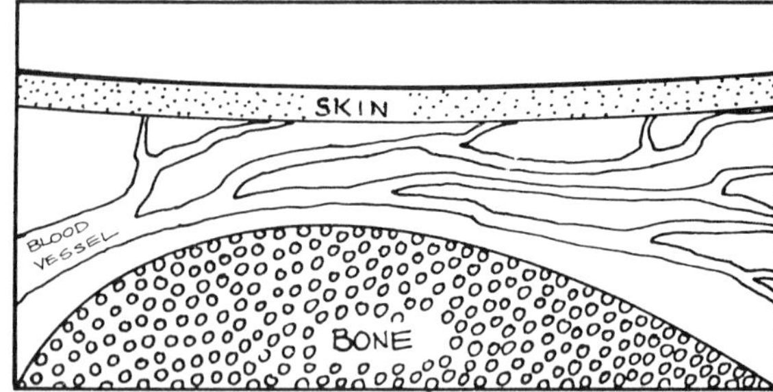

(b) Pressure

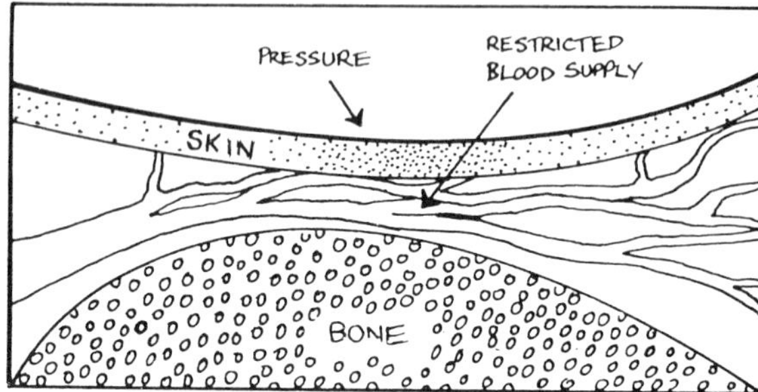

(c) Cell Damage

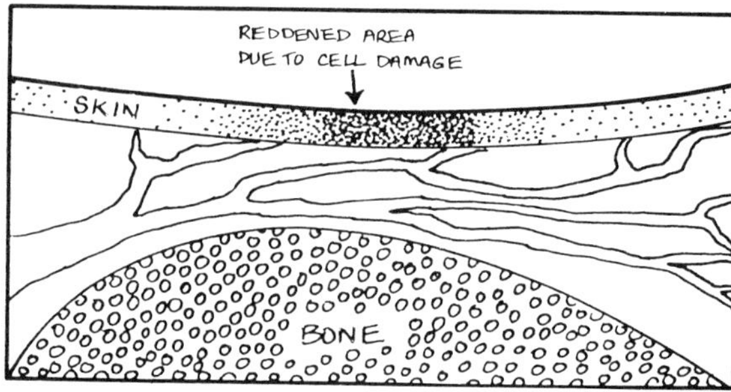

(d) Cell Death

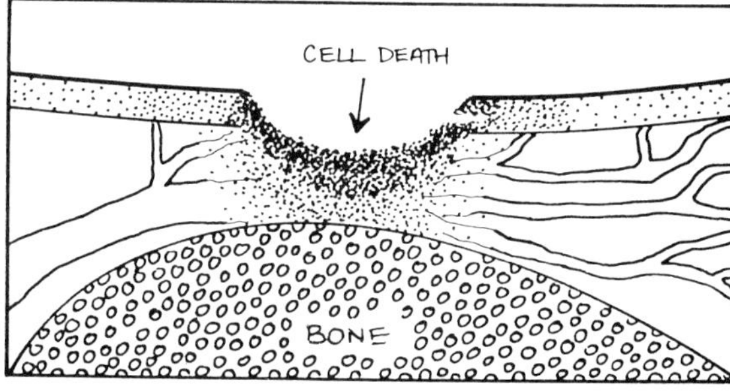

(e) Dead Tissue

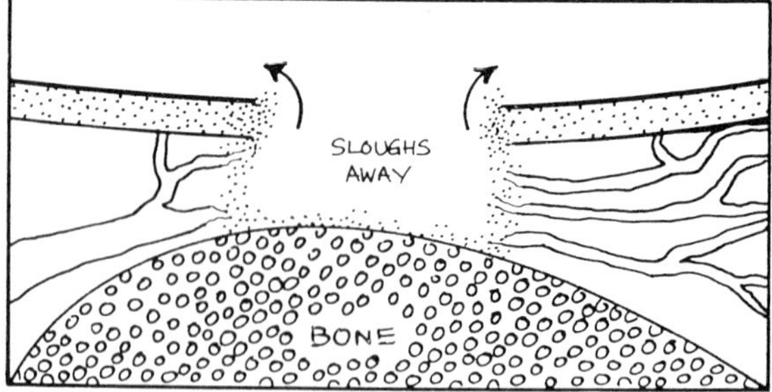

Fig. 2.1 (a) to (e) Development of a pressure area

- all bony areas around the buttocks, sacrum, trochanters (bony prominences at the lower side of the hips) and ischial tuberosities (bony prominences that take your weight when you sit)
- the hips
- the knees
- the heels
- the ankles

Causes of pressure sores

These are the major causes:

- **Pressure:** remember, 'you can put anything on a pressure area except yourself'.
- **Moisture:** ensure you are completely dry following showering or baths; especially watch your groin areas. If urine gets on your skin, ensure that it is completely washed off, or your skin may become soft and easily broken.
- **Tapes:** if sticking plaster is pulled off too quickly, skin may be damaged.
- **Tight clothing:** the seams on tight jeans or trousers will rub your skin.
- **Poor diet:** if your diet is poor, your skin condition will deteriorate.
- **Objects left in bed:** watch for hard things in bed that you may lie on, such as bottle tops, scissors or crumbs.
- **Spasm:** when spasm occurs, the whole body may be moved over the bed, or one part of the body may be rubbed against another part. This can cause shearing stress. Pillows or foam placed between the knees help to prevent this.
- **Catheter tubing and/or leg bags:** tubing left in one place under tight clothing will cause indentations in the skin. Straps on leg bags must not be too tight.
- **Ingrown toenails:** toenails must be cut straight across and kept short and clean. Ingrown toenails cause excess spasm, which can cause pressure areas.
- **Splints:** these can rub on bony prominences such as knees and ankles, and must be watched carefully.
- **Uridome:** penile skin must be washed and uridomes changed daily. Avoid regularly placing uridomes in the same position, as this can cause skin damage from the adhesive and cleaning agent.
- **Burns:** be careful of sunburn, wheelchair footplates in the sun, heaters, hot water dripping from taps, hot pipes under sinks and basins, hot soups and drinks, hot dinner plates, car floors etc.

Things that do not prevent pressure sores

These things are:

- **Methylated spirits:** this is not advisable on backs, as it can dry the skin excessively.
- **Massage:** this may be attempted with creams, soap, water, and oils, to give comfort, but rough rubbing may damage skin with poor circulation.

What to do if a sore develops

As soon as you find a red area, keep off it. Go straight to bed if you cannot keep off it in your chair. If a broken area reoccurs, go to bed and keep off the sore. If it starts to get bigger and/or becomes black or infected, see your doctor.

You must stay off these sores until they are completely healed.

When a pressure sore heals, it does so with scar tissue. This is very prone to breaking down again. You must build up a tolerance for sitting on newly healed areas. Commence by sitting for five minutes at a time, and work upwards from this.

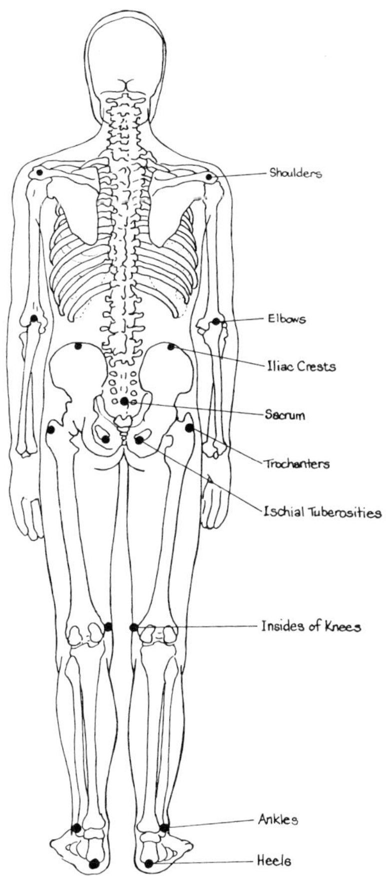

Fig. 2.2 Areas prone to pressure

The bladder

The bladder is a hollow muscular bag that stores urine. Urine is a fluid that contains waste products from the body. It is formed by the kidneys. The kidneys are two structures that lie at the back of the abdomen—one on each side just below the level of the chest.

Urine formed flows into a collecting system in the kidneys and runs down two tubes, the **ureters** (one on each side), into the bladder. Another tube, called the **urethra,** leads from the bladder to the outside of the body. A muscular valve called the **sphincter,** located in the urethra, closes to store urine in the bladder and opens when a person wants to pass urine.

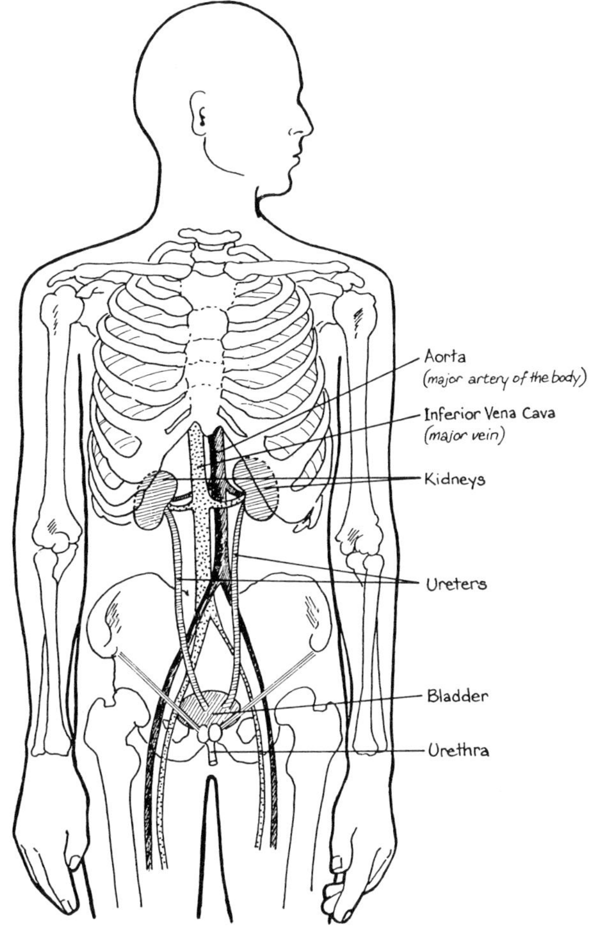

Fig. 2.3 The urinary system

■ How does the bladder work?

Urine is stored in the bladder. Information on the volume of urine in the bladder (that is, on how much the bladder is being stretched by the urine it contains) is transmitted to the lower spinal cord, and then to the brain. As the bladder becomes full, a desire to empty it is felt. If a person decides to pass urine, signals from the brain to the lower spinal cord trigger two responses. One response starts the bladder (which is just a water-proof muscular bag, as we said) contracting and squeezing the urine out down the urethra. The other response causes the muscle of the sphincter mechanism to relax, opening the 'valve' system and allowing the urine to flow down the urethra and out.

Normally, the desire to void can be inhibited or suppressed until the person is in a satisfactory place for emptying the bladder. Usually the bladder empties completely. This is important, because urine left in the bladder can cause a number of problems, such as infections and calculi (stones).

How does a spinal injury affect this?

A spinal injury can interfere with the sending of signals to the brain, and from the brain to parts of the body. If the circuits are damaged, both the ability to control the bladder and the ability of the bladder to work will be affected. The effects depend on the level of injury and the degree of damage to the spinal cord.

Initially, if spinal shock is present, the bladder will not work, and will need to be drained by a tube called a **catheter,** which is passed along the urethra and connected to a bottle.

Often, when bladder function has been disturbed, special tests are required to establish how the bladder muscle and sphincter are behaving. These tests include urodynamic studies, measurements of residual volume, ultrasound examinations of the bladder and kidneys, and intravenous pyelography. (See under 'Routine tests', p.14.) The tests are performed as soon as possible after the spinal-injured patient is allowed out of bed.

The neurological problems (problems of nerve control) with the bladder and sphincter that can occur after spinal cord injury are a bladder that is either too active or not active enough, and a sphincter that is either too active or not active enough. Combinations of the two can occur. This could mean, for example, a bladder that is not active enough and a sphincter that is too active.

■ Bladder management

If there is damage to the control and function of the bladder, a method of emptying the bladder must be found that is practical and effective and allows normal kidney function. The method will depend on the hand function, mobility and bladder and sphincter function of the injured person.

Types of bladder seen after spinal injury

Three different types of bladder change, referred to as types of neurogenic bladders, can be seen after nervous system damage. Two are due to an overactive bladder, and the other to an underactive bladder.

Uninhibited bladder

The person with this type of bladder is able to pass urine voluntarily. However, this control is limited to a smaller volume of urine than normal. Once the bladder fills past a certain amount, the person feels a very strong desire to empty the bladder, which is not able to be postponed. Wetting (incontinence) will occur if a toilet is not found very rapidly.

Wetting can be avoided by emptying the bladder before it becomes full enough to trigger the emptying reflex, **micturition,** or by taking a drug to make the bladder less sensitive to stretch, thereby allowing it to contain a larger volume of urine.

Spinal reflex bladder

The person with this type of bladder has no voluntary control. The bladder contracts and empties automatically by reflex activity. It will empty after a certain volume is reached, or if the bladder is stimulated by activity that increases abdominal pressure: moving, or tapping the abdomen **(percussion).** The lower spinal cord reflexes that empty the bladder can also be set off by scratching the skin on the penis or perineum or anal region.

Bladder volumes that trigger the reflex are lower than the normal capacity of the bladder.

This type of bladder is frequently complicated by two other conditions, called **reflux** and **detrusor–sphincter dyssynergia.** These will be explained below.

Autonomous bladder

In this condition, the bladder does not contract at all in response to any normal stimulus.

■ Sphincter problems

The sphincter is the muscular valve of the urethra. If its action is not co-ordinated with that of the bladder, then several types of problems could occur. Two of the problems are due to an overactive sphincter, and one is due to an underactive sphincter. Reflux is another problem that could arise. Here is a description of the problems.

Obstructive sphincter

The sphincter does not open when the bladder is contracting, and no urine will run out.

Dyssynergic sphincter

The sphincter opens only intermittently while the bladder contracts. The urine flows in bursts. The bladder has to work much harder to empty. As a result, the bladder muscle can become thickened.

Problems arise because of the frequent failure of the bladder to empty fully in this condition, predisposing the person to infection and calculi (stones). The condition of dyssynergic sphincter or detrusor–sphincter dyssynergia (the bladder muscle is also called the detrusor) is often associated with **reflux**.

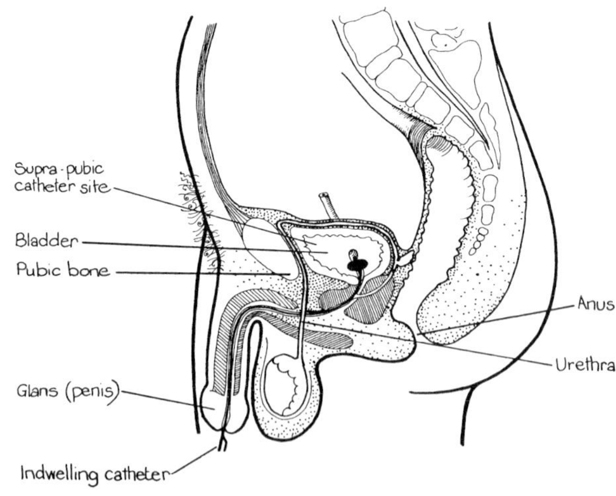

Fig. 2.4 The male urinary system

Reflux

This is the situation where urine is forced back up the ureters. The pressure of the urine being forced back can damage the structures of the kidney, and the urine that flows up the ureters eventually returns to the bladder after the emptying reflex has finished, creating a pool of stagnant urine that can cause infection and calculi.

Incompetent sphincter

The sphincter does not close effectively, and allows urine to leak out continually.

■ Techniques of bladder management

The following are common methods of bladder management. Certain techniques are more suited to a particular type of bladder and sphincter than others. Some require good hand function and mobility on the part of the injured person.

Catheterisation

<u>The indwelling catheter</u>

A tube is passed into the bladder, allowing urine to drain out into a collecting device such as a Monaghan bottle or a leg bag. The tube may run in the urethra or be passed into the bladder through a small incision in the lower abdomen—this type is the **supra-pubic catheter.**

When is it used?

An indwelling catheter is required when the bladder does not contract properly or when the sphincter does not open correctly.

The advantages of the indwelling catheter are:
- It is simple to manage.
- It prevents reflux by ensuring the bladder is emptying well.

The disadvantages are:
- The catheter can block and lead to chronic bladder infection or stone formation.

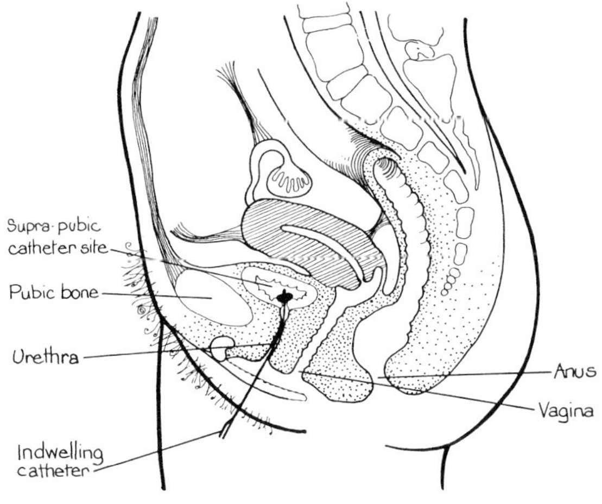

Fig. 2.5 The female urinary system

- The supra-pubic catheter may fall out and be difficult to replace.

NOTE: A BLADDER MUSCLE RELAXANT SUCH AS MONODRAL SHOULD BE TAKEN WHEN AN INDWELLING CATHETER IS USED.

Care of the indwelling catheter

1. **Change the catheter regularly.** Catheters need to be changed every four weeks. This can be done by anyone who has been taught the correct procedure.
2. **Be careful not to pull the catheter out.** Although the catheter has a small balloon at the end of it to hold it in the bladder, it may be pulled out if care is not taken. Always have the catheter attached to the leg or abdomen by sticking plaster. If a supra-pubic catheter is pulled out, replace it immediately as the passage through the skin to the bladder will shrink rapidly.
3. **Ensure the catheter is draining well.** This can be seen by the urine output. If there is no urine output, the tubing may feel cold. The catheter is likely to be blocked. Milking the tubing by squeezing it may dislodge any sediment that has blocked the catheter. If this does not help, the catheter must be changed immediately.
4. **Drink plenty of water,** as this will help prevent the catheter from blocking.
5. **Wash around the catheter site every day with soap and water.** By keeping the site clean and dry, infections will be kept to a minimum.
6. **Use a suitably sized catheter.** A size 18 catheter is not likely to block easily from debris formed by crystals in the urine or cellular debris from the bladder where it is irritated by the end of the catheter. Similarly, a 5 mL balloon should be used, not a 30 mL balloon. The smaller balloon will ensure less residual volume inside the bladder and a smaller surface for calculi to form on.
7. **Prevent leakage the correct way.** Leakage around catheters is usually due to an overactive bladder or a floppy, incompetent sphincter. Putting in a larger catheter just stretches the sphincter further. The bladder needs to be relaxed, or the sphincter made tighter.

<u>Intermittent catheterisation</u>

This means that a catheter is passed at intervals during the day to empty the bladder. This can be done by an attendant, or, if hand function is adequate, by the individual. The technique is to pass a catheter along the urethra to the bladder to allow it to empty and then to remove the catheter.

Usually no external drainage appliances need to be worn. The technique is easy to learn and can be carried out in a chair, on a bed or on the toilet.

Catheters are passed at four-hourly intervals to start with. The person with a catheter must learn to drink so as to have a maximum 400 to 450 mL in the bladder immediately before each catheterisation. The bladder must be emptied as completely as possible each time the catheter is passed.

When is this method used?

This method is used when the bladder does not contract well or when there is an obstructive sphincter or detrusor–sphincter dyssynergia.

These are the advantages:

- The injured person is freed of having a permanent catheter.
- Infection rate is lower than with an indwelling catheter and bladder stones would not be expected.
- Reflux is usually well controlled.
  These are the disadvantages:
- Infections may still occur, because a tube is being introduced directly into the bladder.
- Leakage can occur between catheterisation if the bladder is active or the sphincter incompetent.
- There may be difficulty in finding accessible toilets.
- There may be difficulty in transferring to a toilet and difficulty in balancing the trunk when passing the catheter.

Balanced bladder method

When is this method used?

This method is used when the individual has a spinal reflex bladder and there is good co-ordination between bladder contraction and sphincter relaxation. If this is the case, the bladder works automatically and may be triggered by tapping (percussion) on the lower abdomen. Usually a high fluid intake is recommended and percussion should be carried out every two hours.

A urinary collecting device is worn, the most common for men being a **uridome.** This is a rubber sheath that fits over the penis and is held in place by adhesive. A tube at the end leads to a collecting device such as a leg bag. Satisfactory collecting devices for women do not as yet exist, and this technique requires that women transfer to toilets.

Advantages

- Hand function does not have to be good for the technique to be successful.
- The person is catheter-free.
- The infection rate is low.
- Trips to the toilet are infrequent.

Disadvantages

- Urinary appliances need to be worn.
- Infections can occur if the bladder is not emptying properly.
- Reflux may occur without warning or symptoms

and cause kidney damage, so frequent medical assessment is needed. A regular IVP (intravenous pyelogram) or ultrasound examination of the kidneys is advisable to ensure that reflux is not causing damage, if this method is used.

Special surgical procedures for continence

Sphincterotomy for detrusor–sphincter dyssynergia

In order to overcome the failure of the sphincter to relax when the bladder contracts, it can be weakened artificially. Drugs such as prazosin and phenoxybenzamine weaken the muscle of the sphincter sufficiently for the bladder to empty itself properly. But frequently, the muscle has to be weakened by cutting it. This operation, which is done under an anaesthetic, is called a **sphincterotomy.** The complications of the operation are:

- excessive bleeding
- infection
- insufficient weakening, requiring another operation.

The advantages are that it allows a balanced bladder to be obtained if a spinal reflex bladder is present.

Electromicturition for detrusor–sphincter dyssynergia

It is possible to have a surgically implanted device that electrically stimulates the nerves to the bladder and sphincter so as to control the passage of urine. The device is most suitable for people with an overactive bladder and an overactive sphincter who are having problems that are not being managed effectively by other means. The device can be used to control bowel actions **(defaecation),** and in some men can control penile erections. The majority of people using the devices find them effective.

There are some disadvantages, however. The devices are expensive. Implanting the device requires a large operation on the nerves of the lower spine. The device is not foolproof, and may fail.

Artificial sphincter for incompetent sphincter

A surgically implanted artificial sphincter may be useful for patients who can empty their bladders, are not troubled by reflux, have good manual dexterity and who leak urine because of an incompetent sphincter.

Breakdown of these devices has been common in the past, though more recent designs appear to be more reliable.

Common problems of the neurogenic bladder

Urinary tract infection

The signs of a urinary tract infection may be:

- smelly urine
- cloudy urine
- blood in the urine
- increase in spasms
- high temperature
- shivering

Those with sensation may have burning when passing urine, pain in the side of the abdomen and the need to pass urine more frequently.

Action to take

A high fluid intake should be kept up. A doctor should be called. Antibiotics, if prescribed, should be taken for the prescribed length of time, and not stopped if symptoms have stopped. Frequent urinary tract infections in a person with a balanced bladder are often a sign that the bladder is not emptying properly.

Overdistension of the bladder

No bladder should ever be allowed to become overdistended (too full). The muscle becomes stretched, and then is no longer able to contract effectively. The most common cause of overdistension is a blocked catheter.

However, deliberate overdistension of the bladder is sometimes undertaken by doctors to make bladder contractions weaker, thereby preventing leakage between intermittent catheterisations.

'Stones' or calculi

The human body is made up of billions of cells. Each cell is a self-contained living unit that co-operates, within the human being, with other cells for mutual benefit. The cells are supported by a framework of bones, and are cushioned and nourished by fluid (blood) that is circulated around the body in a network of tubes. The composition of this fluid is kept remarkably consistent.

The role of the kidney is (among other things) to regulate the amount of mineral salts that are in the fluid. These mineral salts are substances formed from sodium, calcium, phosphorus, potassium and so on.

The body maintains itself in balance. For instance, if the skeleton is put under load, more calcium is laid down to build up the strength of the bones. If the skeleton is rested in bed for long periods, the calcium is removed by the bone cells, enters the circulation and is removed by the kidney into the urine.

The salts in the urine are dissolved in water. If the amount (concentration) of these salts becomes too great, or if the chemical properties of the urine are changed too much (the urine becomes too acid or too alkaline), the salts will precipitate (come out of solution). These precipitated salts then build up on catheters as encrustations, or build up on cellular debris to form stones.

Factors that cause stones to be formed are:

- not enough water for the salts to dissolve in
- infections: the bacteria change the chemical nature of the urine and can cause salts to come out of solution
- foreign bodies: catheters can act as a focus for salts to come out of solution
- stagnant urine: large volumes of urine that remain in the bladder lead to bacterial growth, a change in urine composition and stone formation

Stones in the urinary system are problems as:

- they protect bacteria from antibiotics, so urinary

Table 2.2 *Complications of the bladder*

Complication	How to recognise the problem	What to do if the problem arises	How to prevent the problem occurring again
Urinary tract infection (UTI)	• Cloudy urine • Offensive-smelling urine • Feeling 'unwell' • Rise in temperature • Sweating and rigors	• See your doctor • Have a urine specimen taken for culture • Take the full course of antibiotics if prescribed	• Drink three to four litres of clear fluid each day. • If you have a catheter, use an Alcowipe each time you disconnect it from the tubing. • If using other methods to empty the bladder—percussion or expression—make sure the bladder is emptying completely every two hours, as high residuals will lead to infection. • Daily washing of the perineal area, especially following a bowel action.
Bladder calculi ('stones')	• Increase in sediment in the urine • Increase in spasm • Pain • Passing of stones	• Contact your doctor • X-ray will be required • Surgical removal will probably be necessary	• Drink three to four litres of clear fluid each day. • Avoid dairy products and drink no more than one glass of milk each day. • Keep mobile—get out of bed and be active.
Autonomic dysreflexia	• Pounding headache • Sweating flushed face • Increased blood pressure • Decrease in pulse • Overdistension of bladder	• Medical emergency; see your doctor or go to the nearest hospital • Catheter should be changed, or inserted if you do not already have one	Make sure your catheter is draining at all times and that it is not kinked or blocked in any way.

tract infections are likely to recur.

- if they are formed in the kidney they destroy kidney tissue.
- they may block the tubes of the urinary system and lead to loss of function of the kidneys.
- they may cause increased spasticity by irritating the tissues of the urinary system.

Stones may be detected by:

- x-rays, especially the IVP
- inspection of the system, using special instruments

Stones should be removed wherever possible. However, prevention is better than cure. Here are methods of preventing stones:

- Drink more than four litres of water per day if using an indwelling catheter.
- Reduce your calcium intake: cut down on meat and dairy products.
- Keep active: this stops the bones from breaking down too rapidly.
- Make sure your bladder empties properly.

Lithotripsy

By using shock waves focused on the stone, it is possible to break up some renal stones, and thereby avoid the need for surgery. This technique is called **lithotripsy**. The person is suspended in a water bath, which transmits shock waves generated by an electric spark. The shock waves are focused by parabolic mirrors and pass through the body harmlessly, but fracture the rigid crystalline structure of the stone. The fragments of the stone are then passed in the urine.

Autonomic dysreflexia or autonomic hyperreflexia —a medical emergency

Nerves that supply the organs of the body such as the heart, the gut and the bladder are found in two systems. One is called the **sympathetic nervous system,** and the other the **parasympathetic nervous system.**

Each system tends to counteract the effects of the other. The sympathetic nerves, for instance, speed up the heart rate, while the parasympathetic nerves slow it down.

Painful events, such as an overfilled bladder (caused by a blocked catheter) or ingrown toenails, can cause excessive activity in the sympathetic nervous system of people with spinal cord injuries, especially in those with a lesion above T5. This excess activity can cause blood pressure to rise to dangerously high levels. Untreated, the condition could cause a stroke, and this may sometimes prove fatal.

The symptoms of high blood pressure are a pounding headache, sweating above the level of the spinal cord injury, anxiety, a flushed face and a slow pulse rate. The blood pressure is elevated.

The best treatment is to remove the cause of the pain if at all possible. The problem is most frequently seen with catheter blockage causing distension of the bladder, and catheters should be immediately unblocked or replaced if necessary.

It is important to sit up to help lower the blood pressure while correcting the cause. It may be necessary to use drugs both to damp the sympathetic nervous system and to reduce blood pressure.

Autonomic hyperreflexia is an emergency, and should be treated as rapidly as possible.

■ Care of the urinary drainage systems

Uridomes

Uridomes must be changed daily, and penile skin checked for any redness or breaks.

Leg bags

All leg bags and urine drainage bottles and tubing must be kept clean to prevent infection. They should be rinsed with water and soaked in Milton (50 mL of Milton to 4L of water) for one hour every night. Do not rinse a leg bag after sterilisation.

Fluid intake

If you are using the balanced bladder method or an indwelling catheter you should drink at least three to four litres of water each day. A high urine flow helps wash away bacteria in the bladder and reduces stone formation.

Do not drink large quantities of milk, as too much calcium may be taken in and stones may form in the bladder. Also avoid large quantities of citrus (orange, grapefruit) juice and tomatoes, as these may lead to an excess of oxalic acid. This acid also forms stones.

Routine tests

Intravenous pyelogram (IVP)

This is a series of x-ray photographs taken of the kidneys after injecting into the blood a chemical agent that is opaque to x-rays (shows up on x-rays). The agent is removed from the blood by the kidneys, and outlines the collecting system in the kidneys, the ureters and the bladder. This enables the doctors to tell if there are stones in the system, if the bladder is contracting too hard and if there is reflux. An IVP is needed every year if the bladder is not functioning normally.

Residuals

The residual urine is the volume or amount of urine that is left in the bladder after it has been emptied by voluntary effort. It is measured by asking the person to empty his or her bladder, passing a catheter to collect any urine that is left and then measuring the volume of any urine collected.

Urodynamic study

This investigation tells what the bladder is doing as it fills up with fluid, and whether the activity of the bladder muscle and the sphincter is normal or not. It is performed by running fluid into the bladder while taking pressure and volume measurements, and noting any sensations the patient might have.

The patient is asked to pass the fluid back either voluntarily or by tapping the bladder to obtain a contraction of the bladder muscle. The activity of the bladder and the sphincter are watched on an x-ray screen while measures of pressure and volume are recorded.

Ultrasound examination

Ultrasound examinations use high-frequency sound waves to create echoes from the structures of the body. The echoes are picked up by sensitive microphones, and electronic processing then creates visual images of the structures. The examinations are safe, and do not expose the body to radiation. However, the images generated are sometimes difficult to interpret.

The bowel

After an acute spinal injury, the stomach and intestines may stop working for a few days. During this time, a nasogastric tube is required to keep the stomach free of secretions, which would otherwise accumulate and lead to vomiting. Function usually returns promptly.

■ How does the bowel work?

Bowel emptying (defaecation) is normally initiated by the movement of faeces into the rectum. This causes reflexes that make the muscles of the opening of the bowel (the anus) relax, and the faeces is expelled. The sacral segments of the cord largely control this process.

Assistance is provided in the spinal-cord-intact person by straining, which increases the abdominal pressure, and by tightening the pelvic muscles, which elevate the pelvic floor and stretch the anal ring.

Straining can move faeces into the lower bowel segment and set off the defaecation reflexes. These reflexes tend not to be as strong as those evoked by the normal action of the gut.

When the stomach is stretched by swallowed food during a meal, it provokes a reflex, the **gastrocolic reflex**, that starts defaecation. This usually occurs about 15 minutes after a meal.

How does a spinal injury affect the bowel?

Upper motor neurone bowel

If the spinal cord damage, or lesion, is above the sacral segments, the basic cord reflexes for automatic defaecation are present. The loss of the voluntary components such as straining means that the reflexes cannot be started easily. Stimulation of the bowel is necessary, by means of a suppository, an enema, or medication arriving from the stomach.

If sensation is lost, emptying may occur without warning, so soiling may occur. This problem is overcome by training the bowel to empty at a regular time. Emptying every two days is the most common practice,

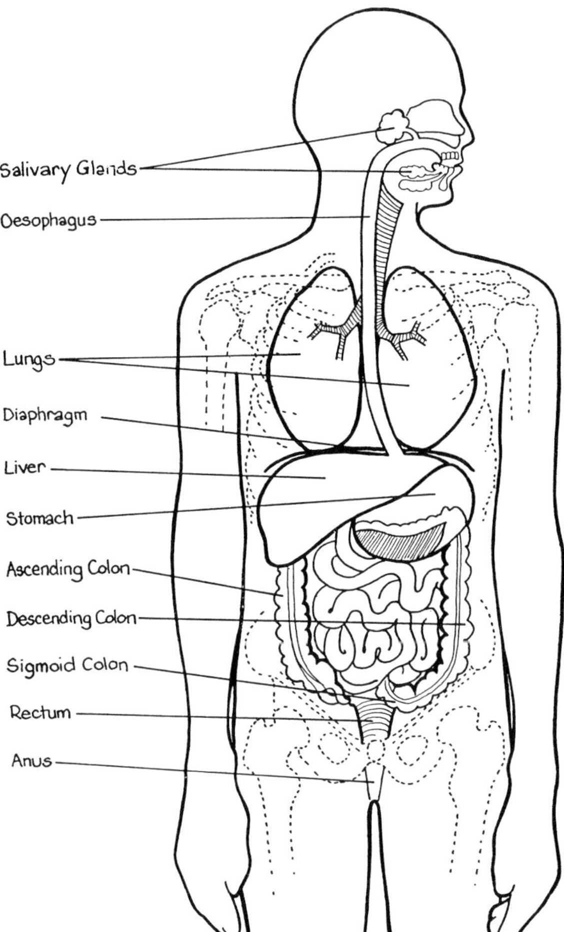

Fig. 2.6 The digestive system

and this is achieved by the use of drugs and enemas. (An enema is a fluid run into the rectum or the very lowest part of the bowel to stimulate the emptying reflex.)

Constipation should be avoided. Hard faeces are difficult for the bowel to move. A good intake of water and of foods high in dietary fibres, such as vegetables, fruit and bran, is advisable.

Lower motor neurone bowel

If the lesion is in the sacral segments or the cauda equina, the defaecation reflexes are lost. The faeces move slowly towards the anus, but the bowel lacks the vigorous motion necessary to expel its contents. Straining by using the abdominal muscles may be sufficient to empty the lower bowel, though in some cases removal of faeces with a gloved finger may be necessary. Constipation should be avoided at all costs.

■ Bowel care

Bowel care is aimed at providing the spinal-injured person with the means of having a bowel motion at the time and in the place most convenient to him or her. In practice, this usually means training the bowel so that it empties at a regular time. This is achieved by:

- utilising the reflex action of the bowel to empty itself

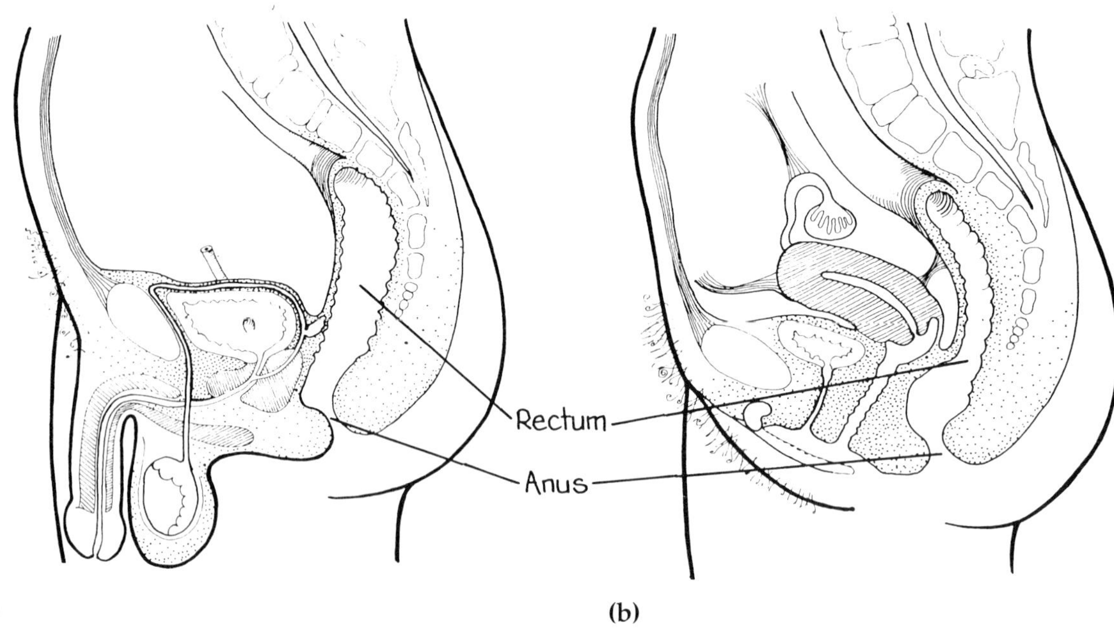

Fig. 2.7 The lower bowel in (a) the male and (b) the female

(a)

(b)

- causing the bowel to empty by stimulating the muscle in the wall. This can be done by:
  - rubbing the anus and the rectal wall with a gloved finger
  - suppositories or enemas
  - drugs taken by mouth
  - timing the bowel action to take place about 15 minutes after a meal so as to use the gastro-colic reflex
  - manual removal, whereby people who have lost the reflex activity in the bowel may have to remove faeces by use of a gloved finger

In all events, having a high fluid intake and a diet rich in vegetable fibre is an excellent way to help maintain your regularity.

Points to consider in bowel care

Diet

- a high fibre intake, for example bran, fruit, vegetables
- adequate fluid intake
- diet adjusted, so that motions are of the right consistency (i.e. not too soft, not too hard)

Routine

Establish a regular routine. This means having a bowel action regularly at the same time and in the same way. If changes are made:

- change one thing at a time
- allow time for changes to show effect

■ Bowel problems

Accidents

Accidental bowel actions are usually the result of:

- a change in diet
- a change in lifestyle
- a change in medication

Sometimes accidents may arise from the incomplete emptying of the bowel at the time of the planned bowel action. This may be due to the stimulation of the bowel wall, which increases the activity of the bowel 'upstream' so that faeces are moved down to arrive at the rectum some time after the planned defaecation for the day. These faeces then trigger a defaecation reflex, and soiling occurs. This problem can be overcome by taking or adjusting a dose of laxative to increase the activity of the bowel so that this 'late' delivery of faeces occurs during the planned bowel action and not after it.

Diarrhoea—'the runs'

Watery bowel motions may be due to:

- change in diet (the intake of alcohol, curry etc.)
- infection
- change in medication
- emotional stress (sometimes a factor)
- impaction

Impaction is the partial blockage of the bowel by lumps of faeces. This may be at the rectum or high up in the bowel. Often nausea, vomiting, vague abdominal pain and abdominal swelling and occasionally autonomic hyperreflexia may accompany this problem in addition to diarrhoea. Treatment involves large doses of laxatives and enemas until the bowel is cleared, and then the establishment of a regular program again. This condition should be treated in hospital.

Constipation

This term means both:

- passing very hard faeces, and
- not passing any faeces when desired

The causes of hard faeces are insufficient fluid to keep the motion moist, and insufficient fibre in the diet. Indigestible fibre acts to retain moisture in the motion, providing a bulky, easily passed mass.

Both problems can be overcome by:

- drinking more fluid
- having more fibre in the diet, such as vegetables, cereals, nuts and fruit. Some patients prefer to supplement their normal diet with bran
- taking softening agents such as Coloxyl
- an increase in laxatives; this is sometimes necessary to help speed the faeces through the large bowel before too much fluid is removed from them

The inability to pass a motion when desired may be overcome by a change in routine:

- Change the time so as to follow a meal.
- Increase the dose of laxative.
- Change the method of triggering a bowel action.

Increased spasticity may cause constipation, and vice versa. Causes of increased spasticity may include stress, haemorrhoids and pressure sores.

The muscles

If the messages from the brain are unable to reach the cells of the spinal cord, and from there the muscles, no voluntary movements can occur.

If only some of the messages get through, the movement will be weak.

Some spinal cells can become overactive because of the spinal injury. The impulses from the brain that acted as a 'shock absorber' or 'damper' on the cells can no longer reach the cells. The spinal cells therefore react to impulses that would normally be ignored. Moving an elbow, for example, may set off a reflex contraction of muscles that resists the action. This undamped, excessive reflex activity is called **spasticity**.

Sometimes a cell will excite large numbers of cells in the cord after receiving impulses that would normally either be ignored, or cause only a localised reflex contraction of muscle. This radiation of impulses causes widespread movements of the limbs and trunk that are not under voluntary control. The legs may flex or extend or shake and the back may arch. Such movements are called **spasms**.

Excessive reflex activity may interfere with movements. Spasms may be so severe as to throw people out of their wheelchairs, or cause sores by excessive movement of the skin over hard surfaces.

This is made worse by any condition that would normally cause pain or discomfort. Such conditions are pressure sores, full bladders, constipation, tight leg bags, ingrown toenails, haemorrhoids, infections, fractures and so on. These conditions should be avoided.

The amount of spasticity varies according to the nature of the injury of the cord, and the presence of any painful conditions. Lesser degrees of spasticity usually respond to physical therapy, especially prolonged stretching of the involved muscle groups.

The introduction of the drug Baclofen (Lioresal) has been a great advance in the management of spasticity. Diazepam has also been used successfully by many patients. Dantrolene is another drug that is less commonly used to treat spasticity. However, all antispastic medication may cause unwanted effects.

■ Intrathecal administration of drugs

Severe spasticity that cannot be controlled by maximal drug and physical therapy may respond to the infusion

Table 2.3 *Complications of the bowel*

Complication	How to recognise the problem	What to do if the problem arises	How to prevent the problem occurring again
Diarrhoea	• Very loose stools • Increased bowel action • 'Accidents'	• Do not take any antidiarrhoeal medications • Increase bulk in diet—bran, fruit and vegetables, unless otherwise instructed	• Avoid any food known to cause diarrhoea • Remain on a high-fibre diet to help produce a well-formed stool
Constipation	• Hardened stool (can lead to haemorrhoids)	• Drink more fluids • Take laxatives and stool softeners • Do not change the time of your bowel program	• Avoid codeine • Maintain a regular bowel program
Impaction	• Constipation with overflow diarrhoea • Feeling sick	• Can be cleared by oral laxatives, followed by an enema 12 hours later. Repeat until bowel is emptied • If unable to clear the bowel, treatment in hospital may be needed, especially for high-level quadriplegics	• Plenty of fluids • High-fibre diet • Regular bowel program • Laxatives • Exercise

of antispastic drugs directly into the spinal canal by a surgically implanted programmable pump. The thick membrane encircling the spinal cord is called the **theca**, so an injection through the theca into the underlying space is called an **intrathecal injection**. The pump lies just under the skin, so it can be refilled intermittently by injection through the skin into a sealed rubber reservoir. A tube leads from the pump into the spinal canal. The advantage of this method is that doses of drugs can be delivered directly to where they are needed, reducing the problem of side effects. The disadvantages are related to the risk of infection or dislodgement of the tube that runs into the spinal canal.

In very severe cases, it has been necessary to destroy the reflex pathways by injection or by surgical methods.

The reasons for treating spasticity are to increase function or to make nursing care easier.

Joints and contractures

The connective tissues in muscles and around joints have the property of shrinking if not stretched at regular intervals. Loss of movement for as little as ten days will lead to stiffness. Immobilisation of joints for long periods may lead to permanent loss of the range of movement of the joint.

Shrinkage which is so severe as to prevent movement of a joint is said to be a **contracture**. Moving the paralysed joints through their full range of movement stretches the muscles and connective tissue and tends to prevent contractures. This should be done regularly every day to have effect.

Therapists may use the ability of joints to stiffen to improve function, especially if there is paralysis of the muscles of the hands. For example, a pen may be woven between the fingers of a hand with stiffened fingers, and may be used for writing.

Heterotopic ossification

Some people develop deposits of bone around their joints after the onset of paralysis. This is called **heterotopic ossification**. The reason why this occurs is not known. The bone may interfere with the ability to move the joint. Drugs to slow down the formation of new bone may have to be taken. Sometimes surgery to remove deposits from around the bone is necessary to increase the range of movement of a joint.

The heart and lungs

The heart pumps blood around the body to supply the cells with oxygen and nutrition and to remove waste products. **Arteries** take the blood from the heart, then break up into tiny tubes called **capillaries,** which rejoin into bigger tubes. These are called **veins,** and they take blood back to the heart. The whole system is called the **cardiovascular system**.

Normally blood circulates through the cardiovascular system under pressure, known as blood pressure. The flow is adjusted constantly to meet the varying demands of the body and to cope with changes in posture.

Standing or sitting up from a lying position would cause a fall in blood pressure if there was not some compensatory mechanism at work. The compensatory mechanism works by adjusting the **bore** (internal diameter) of the blood vessels, the heart rate and the strength of the heart beat.

The mechanism relies on nerves that run in the spinal cord. If the cord is injured, then control of blood pressure may be a problem. People with injuries below L2 are not really affected by this. People with injuries above T5 have an interruption of the nerves to the heart that run in the spinal cord to exit at the T5 level. Because of this, the heart beats slowly and cannot speed up, so problems with low blood pressure are common in this group.

Low blood pressure is in fact the most common problem with the cardiovascular system after spinal cord injury. It causes feelings of dizziness and faintness when the person sits up. Less commonly, the system is overactive and makes the pressure too high. The most common cause of a sudden acute rise of blood pressure in a person with an injury of the spinal cord above T5 is autonomic hyperreflexia.

The problem of too low a pressure is called **hypotension**, and the problem of too high a pressure is called **hypertension**. Generally, the higher the level of injury, the poorer the control of blood pressure.

Tight garments such as elastic stockings and abdominal binders help relieve the problem of low blood pressure. The treatment of high blood pressure depends on its cause.

■ The lungs

In the high-level paraplegic and quadriplegic, the muscles that supply the chest wall may be paralysed. These muscles are responsible for moving air in and out of the lungs. The diaphragm, a large muscular sheet that stretches across the base of the lungs, is responsible only for moving air into the lungs. If the injury is high enough in the neck then the diaphragm will be paralysed and a machine will be required to move air in and out of the lungs. This machine is called a **ventilator**. If a machine is required to maintain breathing for longer than four to five days, a **tracheostomy** may be made. This is a hole in the windpipe below the level of the voicebox. It allows swallowing, and, in some models, speech, while maintaining a link with the ventilator and the lungs.

Very high cervical lesions may interrupt the nerve cells supplying the diaphragm. Permanent ventilation will then be required. If the lesion is high enough to paralyse control from the brain, but leaves the nerve cells to the diaphragm intact, stimulators of the phrenic nerve (the nerve to the diaphragm) can be surgically implanted to take over the lost control.

Weakened chest muscles result in a weakened cough. Secretions may easily pool in the lungs and cause blockage and collapse of sections of the lung, and predispose the patient to infection. Assisted coughing, where an attendant compresses the chest and abdomen while the patient coughs, may be necessary.

Smoking

Smoking paralyses the cells that are responsible for moving secretions out of the lungs as well as increasing the amount of secretions. People with chest wall muscle weakness are advised not to smoke.

Temperature control

Temperature control relies on the cooling of the body by evaporation of sweat and changing the bore of blood vessels so as to increase or decrease the amount of blood flowing to the skin.

People with quadriplegia find that their temperature tends to be the temperature of their surroundings, as they cannot control their body temperature properly. Air conditioning may be essential if the injured person lives in a hot climate. Usually some control over temperature does reappear, but the problem of being too hot or too cold may persist. The brain can sense the temperature of the blood but will not be able to regulate it automatically. There may be excessive sweating above the level of the lesion, particularly on the head and face.

Preventing health problems

Spinal cord injury does not remove the risks to health of tobacco smoking, lack of exercise, poor nutrition, obesity and excessive alcohol consumption. There is no need to complicate a complex set of disabilities by adding heart disease, a stroke or cancer. The following is also important to remember:

- Cigarette smoking increases the risk of developing heart disease, blockage of arteries, chronic bronchitis and cancer.
- The more excess weight a person has, the harder it is to manage independently or to be nursed by someone.
- Wheeling a wheelchair does not normally provide sufficient exercise in a day to maintain fitness.
- Drinking to excess carries the risk of producing pressure sores as well as liver disease and obesity.
- Learning to look after yourself after a spinal cord injury includes learning to live in a healthy mannner.

CHAPTER 3

Sexuality

Most people who have sustained spinal injuries worry initially about whether they will be able to have sexual intercourse and whether they will be able to have children.

For the female, spinal injury causes little change in the ability to have passive intercourse, and fertility, or the ability to become pregnant, is usually not affected.

Despite the changes that occur in the workings of the body after spinal injury, interest in sexual matters is not affected. Men and women have basic drives, which are centred in the brain: to eat, sleep, drink and so on. One of these is the sex drive. Spinal injury does not mean a complete loss of this drive, though obviously there may be physical problems to overcome in satisfying it.

Similarly, the loss of the ability to have sexual intercourse does not mean that there is a loss of the ability to feel pleasure, or to express affection through physical contact. Touching, kissing, and caressing are important ways of communicating and displaying love and are just as important as intercourse and orgasms.

Attitudes

People in wheelchairs frequently notice that people not in wheelchairs make certain assumptions about them. These are:

1. People in wheelchairs are mentally defective.
2. People in wheelchairs are not interested in sex.

These attitudes have to be overcome, and this means having an outgoing personality and a willingness to explore new forms of behaviour. Self-confidence in sexual matters is often boosted by a good working knowledge of the body.

A healthy attitude towards sex implies a respect for your partner. This means being able to share responsibility for issues such as contraception and venereal diseases (e.g. AIDS).

Males and sexuality

The male sexual response can be considered in terms of four elements. These are **erection, emission, ejaculation** and **orgasm.** Each element is under the control of a different section of the spinal cord between T12 and S4.

■ Erection

This is the stiffening of the normally flaccid or limp penis. It occurs as blood flows into the special 'inflatable' tissues of the penis under the control of nerves running from the lumbar and sacral segments of the spinal cord. If the pathways from the brain to the lower spinal cord are intact, erotic thoughts or sexually exciting situations can be sufficient to cause erection. This is called a **psychogenic erection**.

If the pathways are damaged, psychogenic erections are not possible, but an erection may be produced by the stimulation of the skin of the penis. This is called a **reflexogenic erection.** It is usually not as long lasting as erections that have a psychogenic input.

Sometimes erections occur with excess reflex activity such as leg spasms. These erections are short-lived and unpredictable.

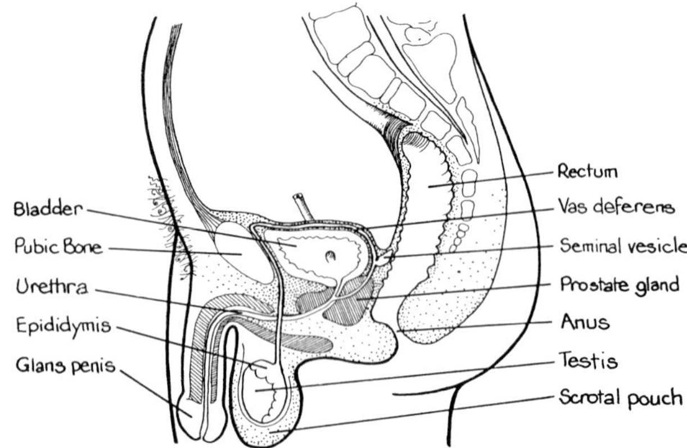

Fig. 3.1 The male reproductive system

■ Emission

Sperm cells in the male are formed in the testicles. They slowly move along a coiled tube called the epididymis lying in close contact with the testicle. The sperm cells mature in the epididymis and then travel along a long tube called the **vas deferens** that leads from the scrotum through the inguinal canal down into the pelvis and into the **seminal vesicles**.

These are two storage chambers for sperm. They lie at the base of the bladder. In emission, nerve impulses cause the seminal vesicles to contract, pushing sperm out into the urethra. At the same time, the nerves stimulate the prostate gland, which lies at the base of the bladder and surrounds the urethra, causing it to secrete fluid into the urethra. This fluid acts as an energy source for the sperm.

■ Ejaculation

This occurs as the mixture of sperm and prostatic secretion, called semen, fills the upper urethra. Reflex contractions of the muscles lying next to the urethra force the semen down the urethra and cause it to spurt out of the penis. The urethra closes tightly during this series of contractions above where the semen enters, so that semen does not flow backwards into the bladder.

■ Orgasm

This is a complex sensation that is triggered by the dilation or expansion of the urethra by semen, and is associated with the rhythmic pumping action of the muscles during ejaculation.

Problems with erection

The erection may be completely absent, or psychogenic erections may be absent, or the erection may not be sustained long enough for vaginal penetration to be achieved. Occasionally reflex erections may occur too readily and be a source of embarrassment.

Generally, injuries above L1 result in a loss of psychogenic erections, though reflex erections are usually preserved. In lumbar and sacral lesions, erections may be lost. Drugs given to overcome spasticity, or to assist in the control of the bladder or sphincters, may interfere with erections.

Penile implants

If erections have been lost and are greatly desired, penile implants may be used. These are flexible rods that are placed in the tissues of the penis by means of an operation. They enable the penis to be bent into the erect position for intercourse. Penile implants may be used to extend the penis so as to make it easier to manage application of a uridome.

There may be some problems. Implants may become infected or extrude through the skin. Inflatable implants, also available, may be difficult to repair if breakdown occurs.

Intracorporal injections

The **corpora** are the inflatable cylinders of spongy tissue in the penis. Inflation and therefore erection may be produced by injections of special drugs into the corpora. The technique of injection is taught to the patient so that he or she can obtain an erection when desired. However, injections should not be administered more than once or twice per week. The major complication is an erection that persists, called **priapism**. Specialised treatment is necessary if priapism occurs.

Failure of emission and failure of ejaculation

These are common problems after spinal injury. Special techniques using electrical stimulation of the seminal vesicles or mechanical stimulation of the penis may sometimes be successful in obtaining semen from men with ejaculatory failure. The semen can be used immediately for artificial insemination or stored for future use.

Collection of semen from the vas by a needle combined with 'test-tube baby' techniques have resulted in a successful pregnancy. However, semen may be difficult to obtain, and when obtained may be infertile.

Orgasm failure

With loss of genital sensation, orgasm is lost. Some people are capable of achieving orgasm through stimulation of other areas, though this is rare. Often a different mental state is substituted for orgasm, and may in some cases be related to the autonomic hyperreflexia that may accompany sexual activity.

Physical difficulties

The higher the level of the lesion, the greater are the physical difficulties involved in being an active sexual partner. There are a number of issues to consider, such as positioning, catheters, uridomes, spasms, incontinence, and physical methods of sexual stimulation other than intercourse.

In order to cope effectively with these issues, an open mind about exploring sexual pleasures is necessary. Many people have fixed ideas about what men and women should do in sexual encounters, and may be unwilling to accept changes in these patterns. Some find the idea of stimulating sexual organs with the tongue and mouth unacceptable, or find the thought of vibrators unacceptable, or believe that it is wrong for a woman to be above a man during intercourse. If you are unwilling to experiment in order to discover what gives you and your partner pleasure, the problem of sexual dysfunction will be almost impossible to overcome.

■ Positions

The positions available for sexual intercourse are limited only by the imagination. Practically, the man would be on his back, with the woman kneeling astride him. This would allow for easy stimulation of the genitals of each by hand or vibrator, and also for easy manipulation of the penis into the vagina. Spasms in this situation do not usually result in any problem.

■ Catheters

Supra-pubic catheters should not be removed, as they may be difficult to replace.

Urethral catheters can be removed if there is a clean catheter to be reinserted, and this procedure is easy to perform. If the catheter has to stay in for some reason, it may be folded down beside the penis and kept in this position by the application of a condom.

If intermittent self-catheters are used, it is advisable to empty the bladder before intercourse, as pressure over the abdomen or sacral stimulation may result in bladder contraction and leakage of urine. Uridomes should be removed after a percussion, or tap to empty the bladder.

■ Bowel accidents

Bowel accidents can occur from time to time. Planning of sexual activity should take into account the time since the last bowel movement so as to avoid problems. To prevent possible embarrassment, partners should be briefed about all possible catastrophes.

■ Cleanliness

Cleanliness of the penis and surrounding skin is important, especially if the person is wearing a uridome, as the moist atmosphere around the penis encourages the growth of bacteria. Some of these bacteria have the ability to break down nitrogen-bearing material in the urine to form ammonia, accounting for the strong odour sometimes noted when changing uridomes. The excess bacteria should be removed by washing with soap and water before intercourse.

■ Vibrators

If erections are short-lived and hand function is limited, or absent, stimulation of the partner's labia (fleshy lips on each side of the vagina) and clitoris by a vibrator can provide pleasure. The interior of the vagina is not very sensitive, and the pleasurable effects of intercourse come from the massaging action on the entrance of the vagina, on the labia and indirectly on the clitoris as the penis is moved in and out of the vagina.

Vibrators that have been inserted into rectums should not be inserted into vaginas without being cleaned.

Vibrators applied to the penis, particularly if they are powerful (80 Hz and 2.5 mm amplitude), will sometimes produce ejaculation in males with severe cord lesions, as long as the lower cord is intact.

■ Rings

Rubber, metal and plastic rings are available for positioning around the base of the penis and tightening when the penis is erect to keep the blood trapped in the tissues of the penis and thereby maintain the erection. Some rings have small vibrators attached to them. They may improve the quality of the erection. However, there is a risk of cutting off the blood supply of the penis and damaging it.

■ Orogenital sex

Many people find satisfaction and pleasure from stimulating the penis or labia and clitoris with their lips and tongue. This practice, which may form a part of normal sexual play for any couple, is a realistic option for those whose erections are poor and for those who have impaired hand function.

■ 'Stuffing'

This means pretty well what it says. It is a technique whereby the female stuffs the semi-flaccid penis into her vagina with her fingers, in combination with rhythmic contractions of the muscles surrounding the vagina and rhythmic pelvic movement. This agitation may often produce an erection, but even if it does not, the overall effect is pleasurable.

Spontaneity

With so many things to take care of—position, catheters, uridomes, emptying of bladders and so on—sexual activity may lose the spontaneity it had prior to spinal cord injury. However, deliberate planning of the activity helps to let events flow smoothly. Difficulty with talking about problems and discussing sexual desires and preferences because of embarrassment can lead to problems. (This situation is not confined to the spinal-injured group alone by any means!)

■ Fertility

For pregnancy to result, a male sperm that has been deposited in the vagina must move up the vagina, through the cervix, along the uterus, and into the fallopian tube, where it must meet and penetrate the egg cell that is released from the ovary at about the midpoint of the menstrual cycle.

This will not occur if:

- there is no ejaculation (no semen)
- there is no egg
- there are not enough sperm
- movement of the sperm is poor
- the sperm are poorly formed

Other factors can interfere with the continuation of pregnancy after fertilisation. Infections, damage to the spinal cord and loss of the ability to control accurately the temperature of the testicles are the main reasons for loss of fertility in the paraplegic and quadriplegic male. In some cases, surgery around the bladder neck reduces fertility because the ejaculate flows back into the bladder, rather than out of the penis.

With current techniques for collecting semen from males, and taking into account those who manage to have intercourse, about one in five paraplegic and quadriplegic males is capable of fathering children.

Females and sexuality

The female sexual response can be considered in two parts: **lubrication** and **orgasm.**

■ Lubrication

Erotic stimuli or direct stimulation of the female genitals produce a swelling of the labia and clitoris, and lubrication of the vagina by a mucoid secretion from glands on either side of the vagina and in the vaginal wall. The swelling of the labia and clitoris and general blood flow to the area are under the influence of reflexes from the lumbar and sacral segments of the spinal cord.

■ Orgasm

This is a complex sensation that is associated with a series of spasmodic contractions of the vaginal wall muscles and muscles of the pelvic floor. Loss of sensation in the genitals greatly affects the perception of orgasm. Other physical stimulation, though, may lead to closely related sensations.

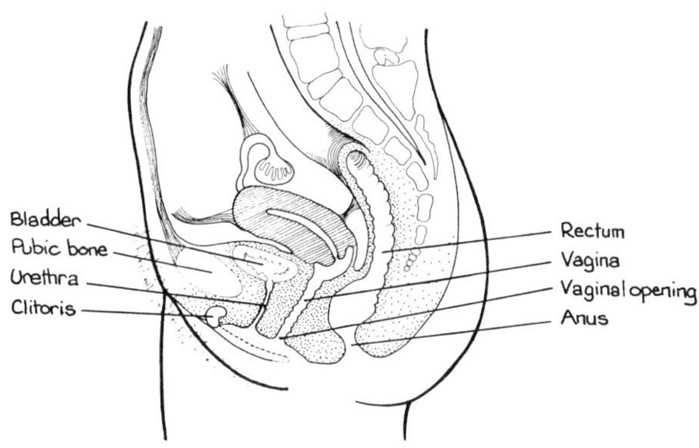

Fig. 3.2 The female reproductive system

■ Problems

Loss of lubrication

This is a common problem and is easily overcome with a lubricant that is water-soluble (washes off in water), such as Lubifax, Surgilube or K-Y gel. Vaseline should not be used as it is difficult to wash off and is relatively sticky.

Loss of orgasm

Loss of genital sensation usually means loss of orgasm. Stimulation of the breasts, which are more sensitive in the female than in the male, may, in part, substitute. Some people have the ability to have orgasms from physical stimulation not involving the genitals, but these people are rare.

■ Menstruation

Because of the stress of accident or illness, it is common for menstrual bleeding to cease for a time. This varies from person to person. Management of menstrual flow is much the same as before the onset of paralysis. Those with good hand function may continue to use tampons if they so desire, bearing in mind that loss of sensation means that extra care should be taken in insertion and removal. It is not unknown for women with normal sensation to forget a tampon that is placed high in the vagina, and this should be avoided by those with impaired sensation. Napkins are more convenient for those with limited hand function or attendant care.

■ Fertility

Women who have spinal injuries are just as likely as non-paralysed women to become pregnant, provided that their menstrual cycles are in order.

■ Pregnancy

There is no evidence that spinal-injured women are more likely than non-spinal-injured women to have malformed babies. Problems likely with pregnancy are an increased rate of urinary tract infection, particularly where indwelling catheters are used, increasing difficulty with transfers as pregnancy progresses, a tendency for the delivery to be earlier, and autonomic hyperreflexia with labour, which may mean Caesarean section in order to control the blood pressure and protect the mother and baby.

If pregnancy is desired, as few drugs as possible should be taken, and infections should be avoided if at all possible in the first three months after conception, as temperature rises associated with infection may induce abnormalities.

■ Breast feeding

Breast feeding will not be possible if sensation to the nipples and areolar tissue is lost. The milk 'let-down' reflex depends on intact pathways between brain and nipple.

■ Contraception

Spinal injury does not disturb fertility in the female, so in order to prevent pregnancy resulting from intercourse, some form of contraception is required. Choices range from oral contraceptives (the pill), cervical diaphragms and spermicides, condom usage by the male, vasectomy and intrauterine devices to methods relying on the regularity of ovulation.

Choice of method depends on hand function, convenience and religious beliefs, and is dealt with on an individual basis.

Other areas of difficulty

■ Autonomic hyperreflexia

Headache, sweating, slow pulse and abnormal rises in blood pressure may accompany intercourse in those people who have lesions above T6. These symptoms should cease on cessation of the sexual activity.

■ Catheters

Suprapubic catheters should not be removed.

Indwelling urethral catheters may be removed if intercourse from the front is desired, and then replaced at the conclusion. A simpler alternative is to have the male introduce his penis into the vagina from behind while both partners lie on their sides. This allows the catheter to remain in position and ensures that it is not in the way. This position also allows the male to use his upper hand to caress his partner. People using intermittent catheters should empty the bladder before intercourse.

■ Positions

These are limited only by the imagination and by the dictates of comfort. Lying on the back with the male on top, or lying on the side with the male in front or behind, are the most practical positions. Tight thigh adductor muscles, the muscles that keep the legs together, may interfere with intercourse from the front, as the legs have to be spread sufficiently wide apart to accommodate the male partner's pelvis. Minor surgery is sometimes necessary to allow this approach. Entry of the male from the rear overcomes this problem.

Resources

Book list

Becket, Elle Friedman, *Female Sexuality Following Spinal Cord Injury*, Cheerer Publishing, Bloomington, 1978.

Gunnel, Enby, *Let there be Love: Sex and the Handicapped*, Wheaton and Co., Essex, 1975.

Mooney, T.O., Cole, T.M. & Chilgren, R.A., *Sexual Options for Paraplegics and Quadriplegics*, Little, Brown & Co., Boston, 1975.

New South Wales Women's Advisory Council, *I Always Wanted to be a Tap Dancer: Women with Disabilities*, New South Wales Women's Advisory Council, Sydney, 1989.

Rabin, Barry T., *The Sensuous Wheeler: Sexual Adjustment for the Spinal Cord Injured*, Multi-Media Resource Centre, San Francisco, 1980.

Sexual counselling

New South Wales

The Family Planning Association, at:

328–336 Liverpool Road
ASHFIELD NSW 2131
Tel.: (02) 716 6099,

can provide counselling on all aspects of sexuality, including contraception, sexual aids and communication.

Details of individual therapists skilled in sexual counselling may be obtained from ASSERT (Australian Society of Sex Education, Researchers and Therapists),

21 Carr Street
COOGEE NSW 2034
Tel.: (02) 665 6660

Other States and Territories

Family Planning Association Head Offices

Australian Capital Territory

Health Promotions Centre
Childers Street
CANBERRA ACT 2601

Northern Territory

Contact your local Community Health Centre, listed in the *White Pages* under 'Northern Terrtory Government'.

Queensland

100 Alfred Street
FORTITUDE VALLEY QLD 4006

South Australia

17 Phillips Street
KENSINGTON SA 5068
Tel.: (08) 31 5177

Tasmania

73 Federal Street
NORTH HOBART TAS 7000
Tel.: (008) 34 7200

Victoria

270 Church Street
RICHMOND VIC 3121
Tel.: (03) 429 3500

Western Australia

70 Roe Street
NORTHBRIDGE WA 6003
Tel.: (09) 227 6177

Other organisations

The Sexuality and Disability Association of South Australia

PO Box 469
NORWOOD SA 5067

CHAPTER 4

Medications

While you are in hospital a number of medications will be prescribed for you. Ask the ward pharmacist about your medication and be sure that you understand:

- the name and strength of the medication
- why you are taking the medication
- what dose you are taking

After you have been stabilised on various medications and are feeling well, you may be tempted to stop taking them. However, usually the reason you are feeling well is that you are taking your medications correctly. DO NOT stop taking any of your medications unless you have discussed this with your doctor.

Supply of medications on discharge

On discharge from hospital you will be supplied with medications for one month. These will be provided free of charge.

Where to obtain medications and what they will cost

Your medications may be replaced in one of two ways:

1. You may attend a spinal injuries clinic at your hospital and obtain a prescription, which can be filled at the hospital pharmacy. Only scripts obtained from the clinic will be filled. Charges will apply for medications supplied; these must be paid on pick-up.
2. Your local doctor can supply a prescription which can be filled at your local pharmacy. Many medications will be available on the National Health Scheme (NHS) under a 'safety-net' scheme (this puts a limit on the amount paid out for medications by a family in any calendar year). You will have to pay the full cost for the medications not on the NHS.

Table 4.1 *Drugs—their action and side effects*

Drug	Strengths available	Action of drug	Common side effects	Other comments
URINARY ANTISEPTICS				
HEXAMINE HIPPURATE ('Hiprex')	1 g tablet	Helps to prevent bladder infections.	Occasionally nausea, rash, vomiting and stomach cramps.	Hiprex should not be taken if you have a urinary tract infection and are being treated with antibiotics.
HEXAMINE MANDELATE ('Mandelamine')	1 g 500 mg 250 mg tablets	As above.	As above.	As above.
URINARY ACIDIFIERS				
ASCORBIC ACID ('Vitamin C')	50 mg 250 mg	Vitamin C makes 'Hiprex' and 'Mandelamine' work better.	Yellow urine.	

Table 4.1 *Drugs—their action and side effects (continued)*

Drug	Strengths available	Action of drug	Common side effects	Other comments
ANTIBIOTICS				
AMOXYCILLIN ('Amoxil', 'Moxacin' or 'Amphamox')	250 mg or 500 mg	Used to treat urinary-tract or respiratory infection.	Nausea, vomiting, diarrhoea, rash.	Do not take if allergic to penicillin. May be taken with food.
CEPHALEXIN ('Ceporex')	250 mg or 500 mg capsules	Treats urinary tract or respiratory infections.	Nausea, rash.	Take on an empty stomach. May cause allergy if allergic to penicillin.
NORFLOXACIN ('Noroxin')	400 mg tablets	Treats urinary-tract infections.	May cause drowsiness, nausea.	Take on an empty stomach. Do not take with milk or antacids.
TRIMETHOPRIM/ SULPHAMETHOXAZOLE ('Resprim', 'Bactrim SS')	Single strength 400 mg/80 mg	Used to prevent urinary-tract infections.	Rash, nausea and vomiting.	Tablets should be taken after food with a glass of water. Do not take if allergic to 'Sulpha' drugs.
('Bactrim DS')	Double-strength: 800 mg/160 mg	Treats infections.		
DRUGS ACTING ON THE BLADDER				
BETHANECHOL ('Urecholine')	10 mg tablets	Used to improve bladder emptying.	Salivation, sweating, abdominal discomfort, diarrhoea, nausea, fall in blood pressure.	
DIBENYLINE ('Phenoxybenzamine')	10 mg capsules	Aids bladder emptying.	Nasal congestion, headaches, postural hypotension (low blood pressure), blurred vision.	
OXYBUTYNIN ('Ditropan')	5 mg tablet	Helps to prevent bladder spasm.		
PENTHIENATE ('Monodral')	5 mg tablet	Used to prevent bladder spasm and urine leaking.	Dry mouth, blurring, constipation.	Avoid driving if suffering from blurred vision. Needs to be kept in the fridge.
PROPANTHELINE ('Probanthine')	15 mg tablet	As above.	As above.	
DRUGS TO RELIEVE SPASM				
BACLOFEN ('Lioresal')	10 mg or 25 mg tablets	Helps relieve muscle spasm.	Nausea, vomiting, sedation, nightmares, confusion, hallucinations.	Take with food to avoid gastric irritation. Alcohol will increase the sedative effects. Co-ordination may be affected.
DIAZEPAM ('Valium', 'Durene', 'Propam')	2 mg or 5 mg or 10 mg tablets	Helps relieve muscle spasm, may aid sleep.	Drowsiness, depression and confusion.	Alcohol will increase the sedative effects. Co-ordination required for driving or operating machinery may be altered.
DRUGS ACTING ON THE BOWEL				
COLOXYL	50 mg	Stool softener.	——	Requires good fluid intake.
COLOXYL WITH SENNA		Stool softener and stimulant.	Intestinal cramps.	Requires good fluid intake.
SENOKOT	Tablets and granules.	Bowel stimulant.	Intestinal cramps.	Granules may be eaten plain or can be mixed with milk. Maintain fluid intake.

Table 4.1 *Drugs—their action and side effects (continued)*

Drug	Strengths available	Action of drug	Common side effects	Other comments
AGAROL	Liquid	Bowel stimulant.	Intestinal cramps.	Maintain fluid intake.
LACTULOSE ('Duphalac')	Liquid	Stool softener.	Intestinal cramps. and bowel flatulence.	Can mix with orange juice to improve taste.
BISACODYL ('Durolax', 'Bisalax')	5 mg tablets 10 mg suppositories or 10 mg enema	Bowel stimulant.	Intestinal cramps.	Suppositories and enemas need to be inserted sufficiently high.

If you have pharmaceutical cover with a private health insurance fund, a receipt may be obtained from the pharmacy and submitted to the fund to obtain a refund for some of the cost. Make sure you do not run out of your medications. If you have any problems, contact the hospital pharmacy.

The table is only a guide, and may not include every medication you are taking. Similarly, only the common adverse effects are listed, and you may experience others as well.

If you are in any doubt about any of the information provided, contact the pharmacist attached to your spinal unit, or your doctor.

Medications table

The previous pages provide a table of medications most commonly used by patients with spinal injuries.

CHAPTER 5

The rehabilitation team

The roles of most members of the rehabilitation team are obvious. However, some do need more explanation.

What do physiotherapists do?

Physiotherapists are health professionals who provide physical treatment. This includes muscle strengthening programs, the retraining of movement skills disturbed by disease, injury or disuse, the mobilisation and manipulation of joints, the application of heat and cold for specific purposes, nerve stimulation and so on.

For a person with a spinal injury, the physiotherapist will be particularly concerned with:
- preventing muscles from becoming tight and joints from becoming stiff (**contractures**)
- helping prevent chest infections and assisting in the treatment of chest infections
- helping the patient build up muscle strength to achieve independence

■ Contractures

When a normal muscle has no working muscle to oppose it or when the control of both muscles is affected and one is more powerful than the other, deformity of the joints may occur.

In these circumstances, the joint will become bent in the direction of the more active muscle group.

■ Posture

Consistent sitting results in bent hips and bent knees, while consistent lying in bed can result in stiff, straight hips, legs and feet.

How to prevent contractures

Contractures should be prevented by:
- moving all joints at risk through their full range of movement every day
- gently stretching muscles that are tightening
- ensuring proper positioning and using different positions to counteract problems
- having footplates on wheelchairs at the correct height so that ankles are properly postured
- lying on the stomach daily to help prevent flexion contractures of the hips

■ Chest infections

Weakness of the chest and abdominal muscles results in shallow breathing and a weak cough. Secretions in the lung may pool and block sections of the lung. Infection may start in these circumstances.

How to prevent chest infections

- Do not smoke. Smoking increases the secretions of the lungs and reduces their ability to move the secretions away.
- Do deep breathing exercises daily.
- Use assisted coughing.

Helping the diaphragm to work

The action of the diaphragm can be reinforced by using techniques to mimic the action of the stomach muscles.

The patient can do this in a sitting position by leaning forward quickly in the chair and compressing the abdominal contents at the same time as coughing.

If the patient is lying, an assistant can push on the bottom of the rib cage or over the abdomen. As the patient coughs, a push in on the ribs and up in the abdomen helps expel air and secretions from the lungs.

The technique is best performed by two people, one with his or her hands on the lower rib cage and abdomen and one with his or her hands on the upper rib cage.

■ Maintaining muscle strength

Keep active—do as many things for yourself as possible:
- Push your chair yourself.
- Do push-ups in your chair.
- Take up a sport:
  —archery
  —swimming
  —table tennis
  —weightlifting

■ Physiotherapy after the hospital stay

This means utilising a physiotherapist for a specific purpose. Most people will have sorted out their own physical therapy programs with the hospital physiotherapists before they leave hospital. Others, however, will need a physiotherapist after leaving hospital because:

- recovery of function is still occurring
- family and friends will need help with physical management
- joints will be very stiff and specialised techniques will be needed for the problem

Physiotherapy out of hospital is available from:

- community rehabilitation services
- private physiotherapists

Outpatient physiotherapy is available from most hospitals and from the Commonwealth Rehabilitation Service (CRS).

What do occupational therapists do?

The occupational therapist is concerned with your independence—with helping you use the movement and strength that you have to perform everyday tasks. This process of assisting you begins from the time you enter hospital.

The therapist will assess your ability in a number of areas, and intervention will depend upon your level of disability. Several areas are covered.

■ Personal care

You will be assessed and retrained in personal activities, including feeding, dressing, showering, using the toilet and grooming. You will also be taught new techniques and how to use aids.

■ Daily living activities

You will be assessed and retrained in activities that include home duties, shopping, driving, communication and environment control.

■ Accommodation

Your needs will be investigated, and a home visit made to assess the need for modifications that will facilitate your safety and independence. Visits will also be made to accommodation alternatives.

■ Equipment

This will be assessed, and appropriate equipment ordered.

■ Vocation

You will be assessed for the potential of your return to work. Work conditioning and retraining will be organised for you, job visits will be made if appropriate, or alternatives to employment will be investigated.

■ Leisure

Different leisure possibilities will be investigated and introduced to you. The occupational therapist, in conjunction with other staff members, will also assist you and your family with adjusting to your disability.

What do social workers do?

Social workers are trained counsellors. They are available to help you and your family cope with the social and emotional effects of a spinal injury. They may be able to help you with personal and family problems as well as offering information and advice about a range of services. Often, when you are in situations of stress or crisis, it is good to be able to talk to someone who understands your situation but can remain objective.

Their advice may help you to understand and deal with better your own and other people's reactions to your disability. They may also help by informing you about benefits, services or assistance that are available in our society for disabled people.

The social worker can help you in several areas.

■ Emotional support

Counselling will be offered on your feelings about being separated from family and home, bereavement, anxiety about your illness and adjusting to your disability.

■ Financial assistance

Assistance will be given with applications for and information on available financial help, such as pensions, benefits and allowances. You will be offered help with financial problems, such as debts, and information about and help with the funding of home alterations and equipment.

■ Accommodation

You will be given information about accommodation options if you cannot go home, and helped with applications to the Housing Department. Home visits will be available, and visits and admission to nursing homes/hostels will be arranged.

■ Legal matters

You will be given information regarding your entitlements, and offered liaison with insurance companies and solicitors.

■ Rehabilitation and work

You will get referrals to rehabilitation services, and counselling about work.

■ Social and community support

You will get information on back-up services, such as the Paraquad Association, the Australian Quadriplegic Association, Community Nursing, Home Care and Meals on Wheels.

Adjusting to a spinal injury

Grieving

There are few disabilities that affect a person's entire lifestyle as greatly as a spinal injury. There is so much to take in—your accident, your hospitalisation, your disability and the effect this has on you and your family, friends, accommodation, work and leisure.

Adjusting to these losses and changes is as much an emotional battle as a physical one. A spinal injury leads you to question not only yourself, but also your abilities and relationships. This happens because experiencing a spinal injury is like losing a relative, or suffering the break-up of a relationship. It is a traumatic loss. It shakes your sense of confidence and raises anxieties about how you will manage and what the future will be. It also involves mourning. When we lose something we care about we grieve at the loss. Grieving involves many emotions—disbelief, anger, sadness and shock.

It is important to understand that these moods and feelings are natural responses to your injury. It is for this reason that the following section has been written. In it we look at common experiences you and your family may have.

Reactions to becoming disabled

■ 'How could this have happened to me?'

Accidents are a major cause of spinal cord injury. Because they happen so suddenly and unexpectedly it is often hard to understand why they have happened at all. It seems amazing that you can be so badly injured while simply going about your normal activities, such as driving or playing sport. It is harder still to conceive how a single event can have such major repercussions on your entire lifestyle.

When you are injured in this way it is normal to recall the events of the accident and try to work out how it could have happened, and why it did. Spending time reflecting on this is often a natural way of trying to make sense of the situation and restore order to your thinking. This process, though, will raise questions and regrets in your mind, and it may be helpful to examine some of these.

■ 'If only I hadn't . . .'

Often people go over and over the events leading up to the disability, examining what they should and should not have done to prevent it. It may be helpful to talk about your feelings in relation to this, but it can be destructive to dwell on actions that can never be changed, and to persecute yourself for what you see as past mistakes. Learning to forgive yourself and others may be another means of helping you to accept what has happened.

■ 'I shouldn't have . . .'

Your parents, spouses and friends will often try to take responsibility for what has happened to you. They may feel that they should have been able to stop your disability occurring. This can be a hard burden to carry, and an unnecessary one, as no individual has the power to control all events in another's life.

Feelings of failure and guilt can be very strong and can create tensions in relationships. Often people try to make up for what has happened in order to relieve their own feelings of guilt, without finding out whether this is helpful to the other person. Talking about these things may help you to understand what is going on.

■ 'Why me?'

This question can provide the basis of much soul-searching as people look for reasons for having become disabled. Honest questioning may be a natural response, but be aware that you may never find satisfactory answers.

Probably the events surrounding your becoming disabled will always be important to you. However, with time, you will find yourself concentrating your energies not so much on what has happened as on how you can go about living with your disability.

Adjusting to the hospital stay and your disability

■ Initial stages

After the accident there is the crisis of being admitted to hospital and adjusting to being a patient and to the initial impact of your injury. The act of settling into the new environment may be accompanied by several feelings.

Feeling overwhelmed

'I just felt numb, like I was in a daze.'

The unexpectedness of a spinal cord injury leaves you in no way prepared for the turmoil to follow. The crisis of being admitted to hospital may leave you feeling overwhelmed, as may your contact with doctors, their diagnoses, and the changes in your body. With all of this information bombarding you, your brain may feel as if it's on 'overload'. The natural response in this situation is to try to block some of the incoming signals. This is the body's way of protecting you. People often say that they feel numb or in a state of shock at this time. This is to be expected, and will resolve in time as you start to feel more able to cope with new inputs.

Feeling sick

'When I was sick, I didn't have much time for anything else.'

In the very first stages of spinal cord injury, many people are often too sick to have a clear understanding of what is going on. The combination of pain, discomfort, drugs and altered sensation and movement in your body may leave you feeling disoriented.

When you feel sick, your body's top priority is to become well again. Your physical care becomes your main concern and as a result you may not want to think or talk about much else except about getting better. Those close to you may need to recognise this fact. You may need 'time out' for your body to heal before you can cope emotionally with what your disability will mean.

Feeling confused

'I was so confused that most of the time I didn't know what was going on.'

After the initial crisis, life may seem to settle into a routine. During this period you may feel confused about what is happening to you. You may feel well except for the fact that some parts of your body can't respond to your commands.

You will start to hope that this will resolve with time. People may be coming and going, looking concerned, nervous or upset, and you may wonder what all the fuss is about. This can easily happen if you have not taken in the seriousness of your disability, or if you do not understand what it means to be a paraplegic or a quadriplegic.

Feeling it's a dream

'I kept feeling I was going to wake up and that everything would be OK. I just felt like I was in a dream—or rather a nightmare.'

The experience of being a patient and being told that you are paralysed may at first be so removed from your normal experience of life that it can have an unreal and dreamlike quality about it. It is almost impossible to believe that you will not get better and be normal, or near normal, again.

'Things like this do not happen to me', you may be saying. You may talk about never walking again and its implications, but this conversation may seem so remote that it will seem as if you were talking about someone else.

Thinking like this is understandable, because your mind is still adjusting to the new situation and trying to cope with the enormity of what has happened.

■ Getting up

'I never realised how hard it would be just learning to sit up.'

After six to eight weeks most people get up and get into a wheelchair. Usually people approach this with excitement and anticipation, as it means escaping the restrictions of being in bed and making a start to rehabilitation.

While this is true, getting up may be accompanied by some negative experiences as you adjust to your new body. Dizziness, tiredness and loss of balance can be problems. So, too, can the realisation of the extent of your disability, which will be brought home to you by changes in the shape of your body, the restriction of your movements, and your having to depend on others.

■ Rehabilitation

Rehabilitation aims at helping you be as independent and self-sufficient as possible, given the limitations of your disability.

The rehabilitation period is a time to test your abilities, work to improve them and make plans for the future. Practically, this will mean working hard to build up your remaining active muscles by loading them with heavy work in the form of exercise. In this way you will build up strength and endurance.

Rehabilitation can be boring and produce discomfort, but persistence can bring rewards. Results are often slow as it takes muscles longer to build up than for them to break down.

Your rehabilitation will also require you to learn how to obtain the help you need from other people and how your body functions. This will enable you to avoid scrapes, bruises and blocked catheters—skills that are essential for your self-care.

A large number of decisions will also have to be made, on matters such as:

- the selection of equipment, such as wheelchairs, cushions, lifts, beds and vehicles; home alterations may also have to be made
- whether to live at home, in a group house, in a hostel, in a nursing home or somewhere else
- whether or not to work, when to start work, whether to study for a new career, and so on

During this time you will also have to cope with your own feelings about and attitude towards your disability. Most people start rehabilitation with great hopes and plans for recovery. Some may achieve these, but for others it may become clear that they will not be realised. Frustration can eat away at motivation. This often happens when your expectations of rehabilitation are too high.

Rehabilitation is not a cure-all. What it does do is enable you to assess the losses and changes that have taken place, and then it helps you to look at ways of overcoming them. It may show up a lack of recovery, but equally it can reinforce your confidence by helping you to master or to relearn skills.

Perhaps the best way to overcome some of the loss you may feel at becoming disabled is to participate actively with your team of therapists in your own rehabilitation program. This means being involved in decision making, reviewing your expectations and setting realistic goals you can achieve, making plans for the future and working hard to make these plans a reality.

■ Being sick

When you are in hospital you take on the role of being a sick person or patient. This can affect the way you act and the way others treat you.

When you are sick you are the centre of attention and concern. Those who care for you will put your needs first and put their time and energy into getting you better. They will try to protect you from stress and worry, maybe by taking on some of your responsibilities and concealing information they think might hurt you, much in the way that a parent protects a child.

By being allowed to be dependent, you can be free to concentrate on getting well and exploring how your new body works. Being preoccupied with your temperature, output of urine, your blood pressure and so on can be part of the process of self-exploration.

With time, your health will stabilise, and although you may still have a disability you will not be sick in the true sense. When this happens there is a tendency to want to hang on to the 'sick' role. This will often happen because a person has lost confidence in his or her abilities and still desires the protection and support of others. The main problem with doing this is that you will avoid taking back responsibility for organising your own affairs and actions. Being sick can also affect your expectation of others. With all the attention you

are receiving, it is easy to fall into the trap of thinking that your needs are the only ones that count.

In the beginning your family and friends may give their time freely. Over a period you may start to see this help that they offer as your right. Although it is not always easy to be the one who has to ask for help, it is also not always easy to be the one who is giving help. Others are going through many of the same stresses that you are, by trying to keep up with visiting, running the household, working and so on.

This can be very emotionally draining, and tension can easily develop. In this situation it is important to recognise the needs of others and to try to find a balance.

■ Weekend leave

Once you are up, and stable healthwise, you will be encouraged to go home on weekend leave. This leave is valuable because it provides time out of hospital and reminds you that you do have a life outside the hospital walls. Weekend leave acts as a trial run, and a stepping stone to your discharge. Being at home enables you to see at first hand the changes that may be needed or that have occurred in your family life as a result of your disability.

It is surprising just how different and strange your own house can seem from a wheelchair. To help you overcome some of these architectural barriers, it is usual for an occupational therapist to visit and make some suggestions as to how the situation can be improved. Most problems can be overcome, but be prepared to practise some skilful manoeuvring until alterations are complete.

Perhaps the most important issue, in terms of relationships with others, will be your dependency on your family. In the early stages you may require quite a large amount of help on your trips home. Your family may be anxious about how they will manage. Because of the personal nature of the tasks, there is sure to be embarrassment on both sides, especially when you strive to resolve problems about bowel and bladder care. The more dependent you are, the more concerned the family will be about their ability to look after you. This may show up as a lack of confidence when they handle you. They may also do things for you that you are capable of doing yourself, and wait upon your every need.

Before you react to this, it may be worth remembering that your family are probably only acting in this way out of their concern for yo u, and are perhaps not sure what you want or need.

This situation highlights the importance of talking these issues through with your family. Although you may be physically dependent on them, you are the one with the greater knowledge of your condition. You will need to help them by explaining your disability and exactly how much help you require. This is one way that you can be independent and lessen the tensions that may arise from a lack of understanding and confused expectations on both parts—yours and your family's. Recognising that your family needs your help and support as much as you need theirs is a good starting point for establishing balance in your family life.

Self-confidence

Each of us has a view of ourselves and our worth in our minds. This view is based on what we think we look like, what we think we achieve, and the sort of people we think we are. We tend to think well about ourselves if we like what we see. However, many of us struggle to feel confident about ourselves even if we don't have an obvious physical disability.

Having a spinal injury will tend to undermine your self-confidence. Because of your physical disability, you are certain to have lost qualities that helped you feel positive about yourself. This may be due to the fact that you are in a wheelchair and feel less attractive. Maybe it is because you prided yourself on some specific quality—say, your physical prowess on the football field—and that has now been lost. Or it could be that you gained value from a particular role, perhaps that of being a skilled tradesman, and you are now prevented from going back to your job.

Losing qualities such as these are bound to make you reassess your worth as a person, and may lead you to doubt yourself. There is no simple solution to this problem, but it may be helpful to examine your thinking and make sure you are not 'putting yourself down' in your own mind. The following may help.

Think about what makes you valuable

In our society, it is easy to feel that worth is only based on what we look like and what we can achieve. The advertisements on television tell us that we can only be popular, successful and valuable if we have jobs that earn us lots of money, are stunningly attractive, or have the right accessories, for example, a sports car.

This is a good time to assess this way of thinking and work out what gives you value as an individual and what makes life worthwhile. In doing so, you should discover that a physical disability does not cancel out personality and character.

Be careful about making comparisons between yourself and others

It is natural to make comparisons between yourself and others. This is common after a spinal cord injury, and can sometimes be helpful. Realising that you are not the only one with problems can help you avoid the depression of self-pity, especially if you can see there are people who appear to have more problems than you. You can be encouraged by the efforts of others, and strive to match their achievements.

However, the danger with comparisons is that they can promote self-pity and negative thinking. Thinking that others have it 'better' than you can lead to resentment, bitterness and anger about your own lot.

Therefore, be cautious. You cannot change others, only yourself. Spending time dwelling on how good or bad others are may use up energy that could be better directed towards your own self-improvement.

Don't live in the past

It is natural to compare yourself with the way you were, or the way you would like to have been. Memories are constant reminders of what you have lost and how things used to be. It is tempting to hang on to the past and keep reliving past experiences as a way of rebelling against the present.

But doing so may only serve to make you feel more resentful, and will continue to remind you of what you have lost. Breaking free of the past will help you to live in the present and plan for the future. Keep the past as a pleasant memory, but do not try to live there.

Relationships

Spinal injuries affect the way you feel about yourself, and it follows that they will also affect the way others see you, and hence your relationships.

We usually take our relationships for granted. However, thinking about the impact of your disability on your family, friends, workmates and acquaintances will raise many questions in your mind, such as:

- Can I fulfil my responsibilities in a relationship (towards spouse, parent, child)? Can I provide for my family? Can I be a proper partner for my spouse? Can I discipline my children?
- Can I cope with being dependent on others? Can I still be independent? Can I accept being helped?
- How will other people feel about me—will they love me, reject me, pity me, stay with me?
- How will others see me—as a disabled person, as less than I was before, as myself?
- How will others treat me—will they accept me as I am, make allowances for me, overprotect me, avoid me, put up with me?

These questions are similar to those we all ask ourselves, whether we are disabled or not. The changes that have occurred will challenge your thinking about how you relate to people and about how to communicate your needs, desires, concerns and care for others.

This may involve learning to express yourself in different ways. For example, you will need to give more emphasis to expressing your thoughts and feelings, as you may not have the same freedom to demonstrate these physically.

Learning to be a good communicator is important because your disability will push you into close personal contact with a large array of people, many of whom you will have to rely on for help. You will probably spend more time with your family than ever before. Many people will visit—former friends, distant relatives, community workers and representatives from government departments. You will also have to cope with the general public's curiosity about your disability.

These situations will test your relationship skills to the limit. In the process, you may have to rethink the patterns of relating that you took for granted.

In the past, you may have coped with anger simply by leaving the scene of conflict until problems cooled. Now if you are angry you may be forced by the circumstances to stay put. When you abuse someone, you may be faced with the knowledge that you will be relying on him or her to get you out of bed the next morning.

In every relationship there is the possibility of misunderstandings arising, and it takes hard work to resolve these misunderstandings when they occur. Rewards come in the form of being understood and getting close to those we care about.

Some basic principles of communication may help you:

- **Be open**—clearly stating your own feelings and thoughts will help the other person understand you.
- **Be prepared to listen**—this will help you understand the other person's point of view.
- **Be willing to work together with another person**—often total agreement is impossible ,but a working compromise may leave you both satisfied
- **Be prepared to admit you are wrong**—we can not always be right, and saying 'sorry' eases a multitude of hurt feelings.

Of course, the temptation is always there to avoid talking about problems because we fear being rejected or hurt by those we love. Although this can be a very real anxiety, avoiding issues often complicates them.

Talking things through is no guarantee that our relationships will go the way we plan, but it is a constructive way of improving them.

Anger

A common response to a spinal cord injury is anger. Anger is a complex and powerful emotion, and the causes may not at first seem obvious. Usually, it is an attempt to fight back or to regain control in situations of attack, threat and frustration. Often, it may be entirely justified, and will provide the energy for standing up to abuse. Sometimes, though, it may disrupt relationships and lead to loss of control in situations. Turned into feelings of guilt and revenge, it can cause unhappiness and pain.

Here are some situations that frequently cause anger.

Feeling put down or attacked

There are many situations that can threaten your sense of self-confidence. Having to place your health in the care of others can be humiliating. Being told what to do and what not to do by a well-meaning spouse, staff or friends may seem like an attack on your intelligence and a disregard for your rights. In these situations words can be good ammunition in a battle to assert yourself and inflict pain on your attacker.

If this happens, losing your temper can be understandable, but aggressive retaliation often destroys your chance to solve the problems that led to your initial anger. It is important to stand up for your rights, but possibly not to the extent of ruining relationships by belittling and abusing people. If you are angry, stop and think; try to find the cause of your anger and address it, rather than attacking and continuing the conflict.

Feelings of anxiety and embarrassment

Sometimes anger is a cover for feelings such as fear, anxiety or embarrassment. The smallest incident might spark anger out of all proportion to the event. In situations like this it can be helpful to discuss your anger with someone who may pinpoint just what is provoking such a response.

Frustration and confinement

Feeling confined or restricted can be a major source of frustration, and this can spill over into anger. Real anger may relieve the pressures and tensions that can build up after a failure to achieve certain aims. Living with a disability may mean that there are always restrictions that will prevent you from doing things exactly the way you would like to do them.

For example, it can be annoying to watch your spouse struggling with some task that you would have mastered with ease in your able-bodied state. The temptation is always there to offload your anger with short-tempered comments that say more about your own frustration at not being able to do the task than about your spouse's lack of skill.

Sometimes we create our own barriers by insisting that things can only be done one way, or by expecting too much from ourselves or others. Trying to be realistic in what we expect and looking at alternative ways of doing things may be a way of channelling the energy of anger in constructive directions.

Suffering

Anger may be a response to suffering. We tend to believe that life should proceed in a certain way; when it doesn't, we feel cheated and hurt by the injustices of life. After a spinal cord injury it is easy for you to feel that life has not been fair, and you can project this attitude onto your family, friends, society, or God. Bitterness and resentment often follow.

We all face the same problem here: there is no way of ensuring that life runs according to our plans. Feelings of powerlessness may only be resolved in time with an attitude of acceptance.

Depression

Depression is an expression of intense unhappiness. After a spinal injury the losses you have experienced may seem so shattering that depression may be a normal response. Failures, or lack of progress, may say to you that you are hopeless and will never be any good. Planning for the future may seem so full of problems that you cannot see where you should begin.

Any difficult or hurtful situations can lead to depression. The sense of despair and defeat that restricts you in your thinking at these times is a more effective immobiliser than any physical disability. Thoughts go around and around, leaving you confused and uncertain as to the way you should proceed, using up all your energy and concentration along the way. Your sleep and your appetite may suffer, so that physically and mentally you will be flat, and too tired to do anything anyway.

After a spinal injury things that happen may feel a hundred times worse than events that used to put you in a tailspin. Everyone, including yourself, expects you to feel down, and there is little anyone can say that will necessarily make you feel better.

You can tackle depression, but you need to be prepared to make a mental fight against the negative thoughts such as 'I can never be good again', and illogical thinking: 'Because I've had a spinal injury, the rest of my life will have to be terrible'. Acknowledging your depression and trying to correct your attitudes can help.

Recognise your depression

Sometimes it is hard to admit that you are feeling down or to talk about what really makes you hurt. But depression is a strong emotion that you cannot ignore, and bottling it up inside you may only lead to greater despair. Expressing your sadness may help relieve tensions that are a natural part of grieving.

Ask what you are saying to yourself

When you are depressed you doubt yourself and your capabilities. Unknowingly, you can put yourself down in your own mind by making negative statements about yourself, such as 'I'm a failure', 'I'm not good at anything', 'Nobody loves me'. Ask yourself if it is really true that you are completely hopeless in everything you do, and that no one, not a single person in the whole world, loves you. Think about what you are saying to yourself and be prepared to recognise that your thinking may be distorted.

Try to do something that will take your mind off your problems

Some problems have no easy answers, but dwelling on them will confuse you more. Going over and over things in your mind will not make them change. Inactivity is the perfect breeding ground for depression. Think about what makes you happy, and open your mind to activities that will give you enjoyment.

Talk to others

Talk to family, friends, other patients, and staff. Get their ideas and opinions, and share yours with them. Usually there are alternatives that your depression prevents you from seeing. Contact with others very often lessens the isolation you feel and gives you hope and sometimes solutions to your problems.

Don't feed your depression

You might deliberately set out to do things that you know will heighten your depression—perhaps listening to certain music. If there is some activity that you know will make you feel worse, try to avoid it.

Try to remember that it will pass

Depression makes you feel that things can never get better again. This is faulty thinking. Time will lessen the hurt and you will have positive experiences in the future. Others have been where you are now and have survived. Take courage—you will too.

Avoid drugs and alcohol

When you are depressed it is very tempting to take something that helps you to switch off mentally from your problem. For this reason people often turn to alcohol and drugs of addiction to make them feel better, turn off, relax, or block out stress and worries.

The danger with using this alternative is that overuse or abuse of these drugs can lead to problems far greater than the original depression. Ultimately the drugs are self-defeating, and postpone your dealing with the problems rather than solving them. They can sabotage your ability to cope by affecting your physical and mental health.

If you have a problem in this area, seek help: things *can* change.

Severe depression

Usually, depression that arises because of an injury is natural, and will go away in time. However, how long the depression lasts will depend on the individual. Some people react more strongly than others, and their depression may be so severe that they simply cannot take their minds off the cycle of gloomy and unhappy thoughts. In these circumstances, psychiatric help and specific medicines may be needed to help correct the situation.

Discharge

Although getting out of hospital is probably the aim of every patient, when the time comes it typically brings mixed feelings: sadness at leaving friends, relief at escaping restrictions, joy at the prospect of returning home to those we care about, and uncertainty about what the future holds. Because so many feelings are stirred up, it is important to talk to others about them.

Leaving hospital is one of the most significant changes in your new life. Since you first became disabled your lifestyle has been centred on the hospital. This has probably provided its fair share of restrictions and frustrations, but has also offered security and time out while you were adjusting to the emotional and physical demands of your disability.

As a patient and a sick person you have been the focus of attention and have been looked after and protected. Being discharged is a break from this pattern. It is a way of saying to you that you are now no longer a sick person and that you are capable of taking up the responsibility for organising your new life as a person with a disability.

Others will also tend to think of you not so much as sick but as disabled, and you will experience the full impact of your disability on your lifestyle. How you cope with this will depend on many things, such as your personality, your level of disability and the support of others.

There is little way of being adequately prepared for the experience. Remember that it will take time to adjust, so try not to expect too much of yourself and of others all at once. After a while you will get into a routine with your physical care, and once this is established you will have more time to think about what you are going to do with your future.

Your carers will also need time to settle into their new lifestyle. It is easy for you to fall into the trap of expecting the same amount of care from them as you received from all the staff in the hospital. Finding a balance between their needs and yours is important for living at home with a disability.

There are so many issues here that we could spend pages talking about the various situations and experiences that you are likely to encounter. Ultimately, the responsibility is with you, but just remember that help and backup services are available should you need them.

Acceptance

Many people speak about the need to accept your disability, but what does this mean? Should you be happy about being disabled? Should you forget the past and start afresh?

Acceptance, or whatever term you may use, such as 'adjustment' or 'coping', depends on your ability to acknowledge that your disability has happened and that there will be permanent losses and changes, but that, despite these, there is still purpose and reason for living. Acceptance is different from:

- **disbelief:** 'I'll get better and everything will be OK.'
- **anger:** 'I won't be disabled—I'll show them all that they are wrong.'
- **bargaining:** 'It can't be that I'll stay disabled. If I work very hard I should be the same as before.'
- **despair:** 'It's all hopeless. I just want to die. It can never be any good.'

Acceptance means saying, 'I am disabled. I am OK. Life still goes on and so it's up to me to make the most of it.'

People can help you along the way, but it is only you who can make the choice as to how you cope with your disability—the challenge is yours.

 Counselling services

Each of us at various times experiences problems with coping with the day-to-day events of life. At these times it may be appropriate to seek out people with special expertise in counselling, rather than relying on family or relatives. The following agencies may be able to assist.

■ Community Health Centres

These centres are located throughout the metropolitan and country areas of New South Wales and provide help with marital, family, drug and alcohol problems.

A list of centres and their addresses and telephone numbers is available in the *White Pages,* under 'Health Department of New South Wales' in the 'New South Wales Government' section.

Marriage Guidance Council of New South Wales

Head Office
5 Sera Street
LANE COVE NSW 2066
Tel.: (02) 418 8800

Other services

The Council offers training programs and groups on communication and self-assertion.

This organisation has centres throughout Sydney. These centres offer marital counselling, to help improve relationships, to assist couples with resolving conflicts, and to help people look at coping with separation or divorce.

Marriage Guidance Council offices in other States and Territories

Australian Capital Territory

Lyneham Square
15 Hall Street
LYNEHAM ACT 2602
Tel.: (06) 257 3273

Northern Territory

Ground Floor
Winlow House
75 Wood Street
DARWIN NT 5790
Tel.: (089) 81 6676

Queensland

159 St Pauls Terrace
BRISBANE QLD 4000
Tel.: (07) 839 9144

South Australia

55 Hutt Street
ADELAIDE SA 5000
Tel.: (08) 223 4566

Tasmania

306 Murray Street
HOBART TAS 7000
Tel.: (002) 23 6041

Victoria

46 Princess Street
KEW VIC 3101
Tel.: (03) 853 5354

Western Australia

755 Albany Highway
EAST VICTORIA PARK WA 6101
Tel.: (09) 470 5109

CHAPTER 7

Living independently

Very few of us can make the claim that we are independent—that we do not rely on others for support or help. What we often call independence is the desire to have as much control over our lives as possible.

Although having a disability may mean that you will always need help, it need not mean that you will have to give up control of your life.

By using services and exercising your freedom to choose, you *can* increase your independence. Knowing the services that are available to you will give you this power.

Medical services

'What will I do if I get sick?' is a common concern of people leaving hospital. There are a number of choices.

■ Consult your local doctor

Your local doctor is often the most accessible person when you are sick. Make time to visit him or her when you leave hospital, and explain your situation. You will then have the reassurance of knowing that someone local can treat you or refer you on if you need more specialised care.

■ Visit the casualty department of the hospital

If you feel you need urgent medical treatment and your local doctor cannot be contacted, the best avenue of help is your local hospital's casualty department. Here staff can treat you as an outpatient, admit you for treatment or transfer you to the spinal unit.

■ Make an outpatient's appointment at the spinal injuries clinic

On discharge from hospital, every person leaving the Unit is given an outpatient's appointment for the purpose of a follow-up. During the follow-up the doctor may gauge your progress and manage any problems that may arise after discharge.

After discharge, people with spinal injuries can use the spinal injuries clinic for the purpose of follow-up, investigation, advice and treatment of medical problems. *It makes sense to keep regular, ongoing contact with your Spinal Unit for the purpose of follow-up treatment, because it has up-to-date knowledge of this area of medicine.*

Nursing and personal care services

■ Community nurses

Community nurses offer a broad range of assistance aimed at keeping their clients healthy and as self-sufficient as possible. Practically, this means that the nurse will work together with you to:

- assess what you can do and what assistance you need
- negotiate with you about what help to give you, how often to give it and for how long it will be required
- encourage you to be as self-sufficient as possible
- teach you and your family nursing procedures
- refer you to other services, such as counselling, podiatry and home care

■ Where can I find these services?

Community Health Centres

Community Health Centres employ community nurses, social workers, psychologists and drug and alcohol counsellors to assist you with a variety of problems, both medical and social. Not all have nursing services, but they can usually refer you to the appropriate agency. Nursing is usually available as a five-day-a-week service, with some provision for emergency treatment on the weekends.

Some health regions have specialist consultant nurses with specific knowledge of spinal injuries—check with your local hospital.

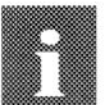 **Sydney Home Nursing Services**

Headquarters:

36 Boyce Street
GLEBE NSW 2037
Tel.: (02) 660 1166

This service provides trained sisters who give nursing care in the Sydney area. Nursing is usually available on a five-day-a-week basis, but some provision may be made for weekends and public holidays. People with insurance claims will be charged for the service.

Local government/council nurses

These nurses are attached to local councils. However, not every council offers this service. For more information, contact your local council. Nursing service is generally offered on a five-day-a-week basis, but additional coverage may be negotiated. There may be a minimal charge.

Hospital-based domiciliary nurses

These are attached to hospitals, especially in the country areas of New South Wales—check with your local hospital. Nursing services in the country may be affected by lack of staff. Visits and nursing care will need to be negotiated.

Private nursing agencies in New South Wales

These are listed in the *Yellow Pages,* under 'Private Nurses'. As you employ the nurse yourself, you have more control over what will be done for you. The limiting factor of this service is usually the cost, as the nurses charge by the visit or by the hour, and their service is not subsidised by the government. People with insurance claims find the service very useful.

 **Private nursing agencies in other States and Territories**

South Australia

Home Nurses (Private)
6 Watson Avenue
ROSE PARK SA 5067
Tel.: (08) 364 4111

Professional Home Nursing Services (Private)
250 Glen Osmond Road
FULLARTON SA 5063
Tel.: (08) 338 1000

Royal District Nursing Society
139 Kensington Road
NORWOOD SA 5067
Tel.: (08) 332 6444

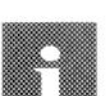 **Private personal care organisations in other States and Territories**

Queensland

Blue Nurses, St Luke's Nurses, St Vincent's Nurses, Community Health Centres and Private Nursing Agencies may be available to assist you.

South Australia

PACS
3A Rowells Road
LOCKLEYS SA 5032
Tel.: (08) 234 5355

HOMECARE Plus
PO Box 283
KILKENNY SA 5009

Victoria

RDNS, local council HACC Services, private nursing and attendant care agencies provide assistance.

Western Australia

Silver Chain Nursing/Home Help Services
6 Sundercome Street
OSBORNE PARK WA 6017

Home-visiting Nursing Service

Contact Community Options (may co-ordinate private nursing and home help in addition to Silver Chain if required).

In other States and Territories, contact your local hospital for details of services available in your area.

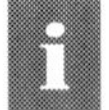 **Home Care**

Head Office

31–39 Macquarie Street
PARRAMATTA NSW 2065
Tel.: (02) 689 2666

Branches are located throughout the metropolitan and country areas of New South Wales. Home Care provides a personal care service to disabled people and their families.

Home Aids will assist with personal care (grooming, dressing, bathing, mobility), relief care, play and recreational activities, therapy and education programs.

This service operates outside working hours if required. The amount of service available, that is, the number of hours, will be determined by the needs of the client and the current demands on the service.

Attendant Care Scheme

The Scheme provides paid attendants who help with personal care tasks such as dressing, bathing and feeding. Attendants are employed by a service organisation that has signed a contract with the Department of Community Services and Health agreeing to provide attendant care.

To be eligible:

- you must be living in a nursing home when you apply
- you must be between 16 and 64 years of age
- you must have a physical disability requiring up

to 28 hours per week of attendant care
- your health/medical problems must be able to be managed in the community by a doctor, community nurse or hospital outpatients department
- you must be willing and able to manage your attendants

The advantage of this is that you have control in determining the service you want and determining what the service does for you.

Application forms are available from the Department of Health, Housing and Community Services, some disability groups and most nursing homes.

Head office:
4th Floor
120 Sussex Street
SYDNEY NSW 2000
Tel.: (02) 225 8830

Support services—housekeeping and meals

Home Care

Head office:
31–9 Macquarie Street
PARRAMATTA NSW 2065
Tel.: (02) 689 2666

Home Care provides a housekeeping service. Aides will assist with essential jobs that the client cannot manage, such as cooking, washing and tidying up.

Any disabled person who thinks he or she would benefit is eligible. Service is provided according to need, and is not refused or restricted due to the inability to pay.

Applications should be made at your local branch office. Addresses and telephone numbers are available—see your telephone directory under 'Home Care'.

■ Meals

Meals on Wheels in New South Wales

This organisation is administered by the local council under the guidance of a welfare officer, and runs with the help of volunteers.

The organisation provides the elderly, the disabled and people in need with a hot midday meal on Monday through to Friday each week. Special diets are catered for. There is a small charge for the meal.

Entitlement to the service is reviewed periodically by the welfare officer.

Individuals may request the service from the local council. Each request must be accompanied by a doctor's letter.

Meals available in other States and Territories

Queensland

Meals on Wheels
Room 425
Coles Building
210 Queen Street
BRISBANE QLD 4000
Tel.: (07) 221 9841

South Australia

Meals on Wheels
97 Fullarton Road
KENT TOWN SA 5067
Tel.: (08) 332 8033

Victoria

There are a number of services available. For information, contact the Community Services department of your local council, listed in the *White Pages*.

Western Australia

Meals on Wheels: Phone your local council, listed in the *White Pages*.

Silver Chain Home Help
6 Sundercombe Street
OSBORNE PARK WA 6017

People Who Care
3 Beechboro Road
BAYSWATER WA 6053

For information on services in other States and Territories, contact a social worker at your local hospital or Community Health Centre.

Practical assistance

Sometimes the help you require may be of a more practical nature—food, clothing, furniture, and so on. The following organisations can assist you in this regard.

Salvation Army

Headquarters:
140 Elizabeth Street
SYDNEY NSW 2000
Tel.: (02) 264 1711

(Branches are located throughout Sydney and in country areas.)

These are the services provided:
- accommodation
- counselling
- transport, or vouchers issued to cover transport costs

- disaster relief
- emergency accommodation
- material aid—cash grants, food, grocery orders and clothes

ℹ St Vincent de Paul Society

Head office:

Cnr Thomas & West Streets
LEWISHAM NSW 2049
Tel.: (02) 560 8666

(Branches are located throughout Sydney and in country areas.)

Services include:
- counselling: information about what help is available
- the provision of food vouchers and travel passes
- accommodation for women and children
- a nursing home and hostel

ℹ The Smith Family

16 Larkin Street
DARLINGHURST NSW 2010
Tel.: (02) 550 4422

(Branches are located throughout Sydney and in country areas.)

Services include:
- counselling: information about what help is available
- the provision of food vouchers and travel passes
- financial help with electricity accounts and water rates
- clothing, furniture

If you own your own home:
- Layettes for new babies are available.
- Once-a-week home visits are arranged.
- Clients are assessed for referral.

■ Organisations in other States and Territories

A list of centres and their addresses and telephone numbers is available in your local *White Pages* or *Yellow Pages*.

CHAPTER 8

Rehabilitation and work

Rehabilitation is aimed at helping people to increase their independence physically, socially and vocationally (i.e. in terms of work). Rehabilitation and work are priorities for most spinal-injured patients.

In hospital, rehabilitation is aimed primarily at helping people achieve independence outside hospital in as many activities as possible. For some, rehabilitation will result in a return to the workforce. For others, it may mean sheltered employment or the need to look at alternative ways of using their time to gain personal fulfilment.

Within the community there are a number of services available that provide vocational counselling, rehabilitation and work retraining, and assistance with finding either open or sheltered employment.

Rehabilitation services

■ Commonwealth Rehabilitation Service (CRS)

The CRS is a publicly funded rehabilitation service specialising in vocational and social rehabilitation for people who have been disabled from birth or by an injury or illness. The CRS works alongside medical rehabilitation organisations. It provides third-stage rehabilitation—restoring its clients' work and social skills and giving them renewed independence. ('First-stage rehabilitation' refers to the acute care in hospital that stabilises a spinal injury, while 'second-stage rehabilitation' refers to rehabilitation carried out in hospital to maximise an injured person's physical and functional capacities—at least to a level that will allow him or her to return home or to some other accommodation.)

The services provided by the CRS are designed to reduce the personal and financial costs of a disability to the individual and to the Australian community.

Eligibility

The CRS can help people between 14 and 65 years of age whose intellectual, physical, sensory or psychological disabilities reduce their capacity to obtain or retain employment or to live independently. Clients are accepted by the CRS solely on the basis that they are likely to benefit from a CRS rehabilitation program.

Programs and services

The CRS is not just another referral agency. It delivers its rehabilitation services directly, using its own team of over 800 professional staff who include rehabilitation counsellors, physiotherapists, social workers, occupational therapists, speech therapists and psychologists.

Additional professional expertise is purchased when it is needed to provide a comprehensive rehabilitation program for a client.

Each client is personally assisted by one of the CRS caseworkers, so that an individual, tailor-made rehabilitation plan is developed, based on the client's personal needs and goals.

Specific services provided in a program may include:

- vocational counselling
- job training or retraining
- employment placement and support
- workplace modifications
- independent living training and support
- modifications to a person's home or access to other, community-based accommodation
- the provision of equipment and aids to increase personal mobility and independence
- car modifications or access to other suitable transport
- physiotherapy
- speech therapy
- personal and family counselling

The individual rehabilitation plan is developed by the CRS caseworker and the client. The plan clearly identifies each part of the rehabilitation program, and details the goals agreed on with the client.

Each stage of the plan is reviewed regularly by the caseworker, to ensure that the client is gaining maximum benefit from the rehabilitation program. The rehabilitation plan may be modified as the program progresses, to accommodate the person's strengths and weaknesses. Continuous evaluation also prevents over-servicing of clients and ensures that each rehabilitation program is cost-efficient.

When the client has completed the program, the caseworker will continue to monitor his or her performance for an agreed period.

Services for people with spinal cord injuries

People who have suffered spinal cord injuries that resulted in severe and permanent disabilities are recognised by the CRS as having special needs with regard to mobility and access.

Rehabilitation programs for people with spinal cord injuries are generally more complex than other programs, and different States have established positions to provide extra support, assisting in the management of rehabilitation programs for these clients.

Details of special services may be obtained by contacting the nearest CRS office in your State.

Costs

CRS rehabilitation programs are generally provided at no cost to the client. Where the client is involved in a workers compensation, accident or common-law claim, costs are recovered from the insurance company.

Financial assistance

Financial assistance is available to clients who are not receiving compensation payments. This assistance is available through the Department of Social Security, and includes:

- a Training Allowance—for people undertaking on-the-job training or sponsored vocational training at a TAFE college or university
- a Living Away From Home Allowance—for people who have to live away from home to attend vocational training

Assistance with transport and accommodation costs is also available.

A large regional network

The CRS operates a large regional network of more than 140 rehabilitation units, and this is still expanding. This network ensures easier client access, a community focus in rehabilitation programs (including appropriate work skills for local industry), and greater co-operation with local health and welfare services.

With over half the CRS units located in rural areas, people from the country do not need to go to capital cities for their rehabilitation programs. Independent living training usually takes place in the person's own home, with job training in local industry and services.

Referral

People come to the CRS from many sources. They are referred by doctors, health and welfare workers, officers of the Department of Social Security and the Commonwealth Employment Service, hospitals, Community Health Centres, insurance companies, relatives or friends. They may also refer themselves.

Rehabilitation units in Australia

There are over 140 Commonwealth Rehabilitation Service regional units across Australia. To find the CRS unit nearest to you, check the *Yellow Pages* under 'Rehabilitation'.

Here is a list of the head offices.

Adelaide

Department of Health, Housing & Community Services
State Headquarters
Commonwealth Centre
55 Currie Street
ADELAIDE SA 5001
Tel.: (08) 237 6126

Brisbane

State Headquarters
6th Floor
Cnr Adelaide & Wharf Streets
BRISBANE QLD 4001
Tel.: (07) 360 2555

Canberra

ACT Office
CML Building
University Avenue
CANBERRA CITY ACT 2601
Tel.: (06) 274 5101

Darwin

Rehabilitation Headquarters
Cnr Litchfield & Knuckey Streets
DARWIN NT 0801
Tel.: (089) 46 3444

Hobart

Disability Programs
State Headquarters
Montpelier
21 Kirksway Place
Battery Point
HOBART TAS 7004
Tel.: (002) 21 1521

Melbourne

Department of Health, Housing & Community Services
State Headquarters
Rehabilitation Services Branch
5th Floor
Westpac Building

399 Lonsdale Street
MELBOURNE VIC 3000
Tel.: (03) 604 4000

Perth

Department of Health, Housing & Community
Services
State Headquarters
11th Floor
Capita Centre
197 St George Terrace
PERTH WA 6001
Tel.: (09) 426 3444

Sydney

Department of Health, Housing & Community
Services

State Headquarters
Rehabilitation Services Branch
1st Floor
120 Sussex Street
SYDNEY NSW 2000
Tel.: (02) 225 3555

Employment services

Commonwealth Employment Service (New South Wales)

Head Office:
Sydney Plaza Building
59 Goulburn Street
SYDNEY NSW 2000
Tel.: (02) 228 9600

Commonwealth Employment Service in other States and Territories

Australian Capital Territory

Level 5
64 Northbourne Avenue
CANBERRA ACT 2600
Tel.: (06) 276 8111

Northern Territory

TCG Building
80 Mitchell Street
DARWIN NT 8000
Tel.: (089) 829 211

Queensland

167 Eagle Street
BRISBANE QLD 4000
Tel.: (07) 226 9111

South Australia

Da Costa Building
68 Grenfell Street
ADELAIDE SA 5000
Tel.: (08) 224 6111

Tasmania

Stock Exchange Building
85 Macquarie Street
HOBART TAS 7000
Tel.: (002) 35 7111

Victoria

222 Exhibition Street
MELBOURNE VIC 3000
Tel.: (03) 666 7166

Western Australia

St Martins Towers Building
44 St George Terrace
PERTH WA 6000
Tel.: (09) 425 4717

Offices are located throughout Australia. Addresses and telephone numbers are listed in the 'Commonwealth' section of the *White Pages*. This service operates as an employment finder.

Services

Special Employment Officer

This person is specifically employed to help disabled people obtain work.

Referral for further training

Officers can refer people for appropriate training courses and programs.

NADOW—New South Wales Association for Disabled Office Workers

10–16 Albany Street
ST LEONARDS NSW 2065
Tel.: (02) 43 0303

This association was formed to help the disabled find employment in the clerical field. It provides, in the form of a work program, an opportunity for on-the-job training in general office procedures, graphic arts and computer programming.

Active Job Services

31–39 Macquarie Street
PARRAMATTA NSW 2065
Tel.: (02) 635 6300

This is a free employment service that assists disabled people with finding employment. Vocational counsellors interview applicants and advise them when positions become available.

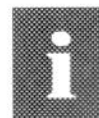 ## Careers Reference Centre

This centre acts as a library on careers by providing information (in print, on film and on video tape) on jobs and courses of study available in Australia.

Australian Capital Territory

Ground Floor
Melbourne Building
Cnr London Circuit & West Row
CANBERRA ACT 2600
Tel.: (06) 248 7766

New South Wales

1st Floor
118 George Street
Railway Square
SYDNEY NSW 2000
Tel.: (02) 201 1122

Northern Territory

Sturt House
15 Scatturchio Street
CASUARINA NT 0810
Tel.: (089) 20 5311

Queensland

Ground Floor
280 Adelaide Street
BRISBANE QLD 4000

2520 Gold Coast Highway
MERMAID BEACH QLD 4218
Tel.: (075) 72 5400

South Australia

Ground Floor
Commonwealth Centre
55 Currie Street
ADELAIDE SA 5000
Tel.: (08) 231 9966

Tasmania

83–85 Macquarie Street
HOBART TAS 7000
Tel.: (002) 20 7100

Victoria

368 Elizabeth Street
MELBOURNE VIC 3000
Tel.: (03) 663 8466

Western Australia

Tel.: (09) 425 4670

For further assistance with career guidance, counselling and assessment services, check your local *Yellow Pages* under 'Vocational Guidance'.

CHAPTER 9

Accommodation

Everyone needs a place to live, somewhere to call his or her home. Being assured of having a home is basic to a sense of security and wellbeing.

However, for a person with a spinal injury, this security may be threatened. It may not be possible for a physically dependent person to live on his or her own. If there is no carer available, the injured person may have to consider institutional care. The physical outlay or location of the home may also be a factor. An upstairs unit, for example, may mean a move is essential.

In an effort to help you think through your situation, we have outlined a number of questions that people often ask about accommodation. The answers will, we hope, make you aware of the options available to you.

Can I live at home?

Most people with spinal injuries return to live with their families, either in their old accommodation or in a new, more accessible home. Some live independently. Where you will live is a decision only you and your family can make. Important considerations are the extent of your injury and the amount of care required.

Can I get help with my care?

Often people feel that they and their families have to manage on their own. However, this is not the case, as there are a range of community services to help the disabled live with their families and friends. These include community nursing and home care.

Is my accommodation wheelchair-accessible?

A basic factor to consider when going home is whether or not your accommodation is suitable for a wheelchair. Key areas to check are entrances, bathrooms and toilets. For help in assessment of your home, the following people are worth consulting.

■ The occupational therapist

Your occupational therapist is trained to assess your living situation and offer suggestions about making your home more accessible. It is usual for the therapist to visit your home while you are in hospital, and then discuss with you what alterations will be necessary.

ℹ Builders/architects in New South Wales

There are builders and architects who are experienced in alterations for disabled people. Contact:

> Master Builders' Association of New South Wales
> 52 Parramatta Road
> FOREST LODGE NSW 2037
> Tel.: (02) 660 7188

This group can give you the names of local builders within a particular area who can advise you on drawing up plans and making alterations. Also contact:

> Architects Advisory Service
> 3 Manning Street
> POTTS POINT NSW 2011
> Tel.: (02) 356 3122

This organisation offers a renovation service. For a set price, an architect will inspect a property and make suggestions about improving its accessibility. Several architects attached to this service are members of ACROD, and are aware of the needs of disabled people.

■ Builders in other States and Territories

Occupational therapists in your Spinal Injuries Unit or in spinal injuries support organisations may be able to recommend builders and service providers who can advise you on and carry out home modifications.

■ Independent Living Centres

These centres may offer equipment and advice regarding home modifications. The following is a list of the head offices.

<u>**Australian Capital Territory**</u>

24 Parkinson Street
WESTON ACT 2611
Tel.: (06) 287 1644
Fax: (06) 287 1640

<u>**New South Wales**</u>

600 Victoria Road
(PO Box 706)
RYDE NSW 2112
Tel.: (02) 808 2233
Direct information line: (02) 808 1477
Fax: (02) 809 7132

<u>**New Zealand**</u>

14 Erson Avenue
Royal Oak
AUCKLAND NEW ZEALAND
Tel.: (64) (9) 65 8067

<u>**Queensland**</u>

Ward 1
Greenslopes Hospital
GREENSLOPES QLD 4120
Tel.: (07) 394 7471
Fax: (07) 394 1013

<u>**South Australia**</u>

180 Daws Road
DAW PARK SA 5041
Tel.: (08) 276 3455
Fax: (08) 276 7417

<u>**Victoria**</u>

52 Thistlethwaite Street
(PO Box 88)
SOUTH MELBOURNE VIC 3205
Tel.: (03) 690 9177
Fax: (03) 696 1956

<u>**Western Australia**</u>

3 Lemnos Street
SHENTON PARK WA 6008
Tel.: (09) 382 2011
Fax: (09) 382 7351

■ Literature

There is a book available from the Standards Association entitled *Design Rules for Access by the Disabled*. (This can be obtained through the Paraplegic and Quadriplegic Association of New South Wales, at a small cost.)

Can I get financial assistance with home alterations?

There is no universal scheme for assisting people financially with home alterations. However, there are some schemes, that we mention below, that may be of help. You might like to discuss them with a social worker or occupational therapist.

■ Department of Housing

If you live in Department of Housing accommodation, your home will be assessed and basic alterations will be carried out. If your present home is unsuitable, the Department will find you somewhere more appropriate. Consult your local office. The social worker will help.

■ Commonwealth Rehabilitation Service (CRS)

People undertaking a rehabilitation program with this Service may be eligible for help with home modifications. For further information, consult the CRS.

■ Home Modification Scheme

This Scheme is for people with disabilities, the frail aged and their carers. It is funded by the Home and Community Care (HACC) Program, a joint Commonwealth–State initiative, and administered by the New South Wales Department of Housing with assistance from the Department of Health.

If you are eligible for assistance, the Scheme may help you by modifying your home to make it easier to live in. Changes may include ramps, rails and modifications to your bathroom or toilet, kitchen etc.

You can make an application by writing to or telephoning the HACC officer at your nearest Department of Housing Regional Office, or calling the Housing Advisory Service.

■ Program of Aids to Disabled Persons (PADP) scheme

In its initial guidelines this scheme stated that it offered some help with home alterations. In practice, obtaining funding is extremely difficult. Your local hospital will have the details.

■ Service clubs

Community service clubs such as Lions and Apex sometimes assist people with home modifications as part of a special project. Approaches may be made directly or with the help of your social worker.

■ Compensation

If you have a workers compensation or third party compensation claim or are covered by WorkCover or Compulsory Third Party Insurance (CTP Insurance), it may be possible for you to obtain money for more modifications on the strength of your claim.

Veterans Affairs in New South Wales

Applications can be made to:

Domiciliary Support Section
Building 113
Repatriation General Hospital
CONCORD NSW 2137
Tel.: (02) 736 6016

Anyone on Repatriation Benefits is eligible to apply, although wives of living members are excluded.

Sydney

Veterans Affairs
300 Elizabeth Street
SYDNEY NSW 2000
Tel.: (02) 213 7777

Newcastle

Ground Floor
GIO Building
400 Hunter Street
NEWCASTLE NSW 2300
Tel.: (049) 26 2733

Wollongong

43 Burreli Street
WOLLONGONG NSW 2500
Tel.: (042) 26 0190

Veterans Affairs in other States and Territories

Contact your Veterans Affairs Head Office for more details.

Australian Capital Territory

Ground Floor
The Drake Centre
Cnr Moore and Rudd Streets
CANBERRA ACT 2600
Tel.: (06) 267 1411

Queensland

133 Mary Street
BRISBANE QLD 4000
Tel.: (07) 22 38333

and

Cnr Walker & Stanley Streets
TOWNSVILLE QLD 4810
Tel.: (077) 22 3333

South Australia

Adelaide House
55 Waymouth Street
ADELAIDE SA 5000
Tel.: (08) 213 2611

Tasmania

Kirksway House
6 Kirksway Place
HOBART TAS 7000
Tel.: (002) 21 6666

Victoria

300 Latrobe Street
MELBOURNE VIC 3000
Tel.: (03) 284 6000

Can I get cheaper accommodation if I'm on a low income?

Many people on low incomes apply to the Department of Housing for assistance with accommodation. The head office is located at:

Department of Housing
23 Moore Street
LIVERPOOL NSW 2170
Tel.: (02) 821 6111

The Department aims to provide low-cost accommodation for people with a low income—there is a means test on income. Accommodation is provided throughout New South Wales, and is also available to disabled people in single and family units.

■ Applications

Applications for permanent accommodation may be made to your local office. These are listed in the 'New South Wales Government' section of the *White Pages*, under 'Department of Housing of New South Wales'.

If you apply to the Priority Housing Committee you can ask that your application be give special priority, enabling you to jump the waiting list. When you present your application, it may be helpful to have a supporting letter from your doctor and/or social worker.

What if I cannot return to live with my family?

For many reasons some people will not be able to return to their previous accommodation or live with their families. In these cases there are a number of alternatives to consider.

■ Independent houses

Many of these households are being established under the auspices of organisations representing disabled people. Here are some examples.

Total Living Foundation

Total Living Foundation
186 Livingstone Road
MARRICKVILLE NSW 2204
Tel.: (02) 569 0643

The Foundation runs four group households for disabled people. Residents share household tasks according to their disabilities, and manage their own affairs. Rent is set at one-third of the pension, and covers basic running costs such as electricity and water bills.

The Houses are located in Petersham, Willoughby, Lane Cove, Glebe, Five Dock and Marrickville. The Foundation is keen to help other groups of people set up similar households. All enquiries should be directed to the Project Development Officer.

AQA

AQA has leased from the Department of Housing some accommodation facilities built especially for disabled people. They include:

Stuart House

65 New Orleans Crescent
MAROUBRA NSW 2035

People with various disabilities may be considered for admission, but they must display an ability to maintain themselves independently. Home care can be organised.

Applications should be directed to:

Accommodation Services Officer
1 Jennifer Street
LITTLE BAY NSW 2036
Tel.: (02) 661 8855

Paraplegic and Quadriplegic Association of New South Wales

Berala Housing Project

The Association offers a complex of short-term accommodation for people undergoing a rehabilitation program. Housing is five self-contained units, four two-bedroom units and two three-bedroom units.

For more information, contact:

The Berala Co-ordinator
Tel.: (02) 749 1255

The Australian Quadriplegic Association (AQA) and the Paraplegic and Quadriplegic Association of New South Wales are hoping to sponsor more of this type of accommodation in association with the Department of Housing. For more information, contact these organisations.

ℹ Hostel accommodation

Kimberly Lodge

This is administered by AQA:

1296 Anzac Parade
CHIFLEY NSW 2036
Tel.: (02) 661 2411

This is nine-bedroom, boarding-house-type accommodation that accommodates permanent residents and has one bed maintained as a visitor's bed. People with all levels of disability will be considered, but must be able to maintain themselves independently. Staffing is provided by the Home Care Association of New South Wales and the residents themselves, with some assistance by AQA.

Applications should be directed to:

Accommodation Services Officer, AQA
1 Jennifer Street
LITTLE BAY NSW 2036
Tel.: (02) 661 8855

■ Nursing homes

The following nursing homes cater for people with spinal injuries. They offer both permanent accommodation and short-term holiday accommodation.

Ferguson Lodge

This is a modern 42-bed nursing home in the grounds of Lidcombe Hospital, run by the Paraplegic and Quadriplegic Association of New South Wales. It offers 38 permanent and four temporary beds to people with spinal injuries. It also offers physiotherapy and occupational therapy to assist with each individual's ongoing rehabilitation and recreational needs. A bus provides transport for social outings organised through the Lodge, which are for either groups or individuals. Send applications to:

The Director of Nursing
Ferguson Lodge
Joseph Street
LIDCOMBE NSW 2141
Tel.: (02) 646 3711

ℹ Accommodation in States and Territories other than New South Wales

Queensland

Para-Villa
PO Box 1377
MACKAY QLD 4740

Catholic Social Welfare (7 supported houses)
Suite 4
3 Zamia Street
SUNNYBROOK QLD 4305
Tel.: (07) 345 7926

South Australia

There are two private houses, Clovelly Park and Thebaston, with wheelchair-accessible respite and emergency accommodation, and 24-hour care. They are run by PACS, with its office at:

3A Rowells Road
LOCKLEYS SA 5032

PARQUA Housing Co-operative provides accommodation. For information, contact:

The Housing Officer
PQA
Tel.: (08) 268 8666

Victoria

The Paraquad Association operates five unsupported group homes for short-term or medium-term stays as well as the Yarrame Quadriplegic Centre, for respite and long-term care. Information available from:

Paraquad
Tel.: (03) 819 4055

Also contact:
St Jude's Private Nursing Home
Tel.: (03) 569 7814

and

Austin Hospital Transitional Living Program
(to be opened mid-1992)
Tel.: (03) 450 5111

Western Australia

Quad Centre (respite and permanent care), run by:

The Paraquad Association
Selby Street
SHENTON PARK WA 6008

CHAPTER 10

Finances

Although money can never compensate for a spinal cord injury, it at least gives the individual the resources to create an environment in which he or she can be as independent as possible.

Unfortunately, in New South Wales financial security is not assured for the person with a spinal injury. Often such security is tied to an individual's entitlement to compensation. Those with claims may receive large sums of money, while those with no claims need to rely on employment or income from government pensions and allowances. So, while different people may have the same needs, there may be a major inequality in the financial resources with which each has to manage.

Those of you with compensation claims can feel fairly secure in the fact that, should you win your case, you will have adequate money available to cover your needs. However, the main problem with this system is the delay in obtaining the money. Uncertainty during this waiting period can be a source of distress, especially if there are fears that the compensation will not be adequate.

Knowing that a certain amount of money must last you a lifetime can be a sobering thought. As a hedge against this anxiety, seek advice on how to handle your money wisely so as to ensure that you have enough for your future needs.

There are many advisors available. These include bankers, accountants and investment consultants. Deciding whom to consult can be a task in itself. A course on money management may give you a better understanding as to who would suit, or equip you with the skills to make your own judgments.

If you do not have the backup of a compensation claim, then it is important to be aware of the government's schemes for assisting you. Money worries can be a great source of stress, and may add to other problems by creating barriers and limiting choices. Allowing problems of this nature to slide often only makes them worse.

If you are in financial difficulties and don't know where to turn, then it might be of help to contact a social worker, or one of the community agencies that offer advice. To inform you about the range of financial assistance available, we have compiled the following list.

Government pensions and benefits

The Commonwealth government provides a variety of income relief payments to many people in the community. Most payments are income tested and have fringe benefits attached. These include the following.

■ Payments by the Department of Social Security

The Department has offices throughout Australia. For more information, look in your telephone directory under 'Commonwealth'.

Sickness allowance

This is for people who are unable to work because of temporary illness or injury from an accident. Your entitlement depends on your age, your dependants, the amount of income you are receiving and your resident status in Australia. A supplementary allowance may be paid if you rent or board. Fringe benefits, such as medical, hospital and ambulance cover, are also available.

Applications are available from your local Social Security Office. You will need to submit with your claim form a doctor's certificate stating the period in which you will be unable to work, a medical details module, identification, your tax file number, your bank account details and your spouse's income.

Disability support pension

This is a pension paid to people over 16 years of age who are either permanently blind or permanently unfit for work due to some physical or mental disability. Your eligibility depends upon your disability, the number of dependants you have, the income you are receiving and your resident status in Australia. The amount of the benefit is adjusted at regular intervals. There is an income and assets test, but this is more flexible than the one applied for Sickness Allowance.

Depending on your income, you may be entitled to a Pension Health Benefits Card, which allows you access to a range of services such as subsidised health care, subsidised pharmaceutical goods and various discounts in areas such as telephone rentals, transport and rates.

Carer's pension

Your spouse, relative or carer (the latter need not be a relative) may be entitled to a pension in his or her own right. The extent of the pension granted depends on the degree of care needed by the disabled or ill person. Medical evidence must be presented to the Department of Social Security when applying for a carer's pension. A doctor is required to complete a form that indicates the degree of care required. The applicant also completes a form specifying the type of care given—for example, washing, cooking and cleaning.

Applications can be made through your local Social Security office. You will be interviewed and your financial eligibility will be taken into account by officers of the Department.

■ Payments by the Department of Veterans Affairs

Head office:

> 300 Elizabeth Street
> SYDNEY NSW 2000
> Tel.: (02) 213 7777

This department administers a wide range of pensions and benefits to ex-servicemen.

Disability pensions

These are paid to veterans who have an incapacity that has been accepted as being related to, contributed to or aggravated by war service.

There are three main classes of disability pensions:

- general rate (10–100%), according to the degree of disability
- intermediate rate, payable if a veteran, because of the severity of his incapacity, is only able to work part-time or intermittently
- special rate, payable to a veteran who is totally and permanently incapacitated and as such can not work

Benefits may include hospital and medical treatment, allowances for wives and children and so on. As allowances depend upon your eligibility, it would be best to contact the Department for further information.

Applications may be made at branch offices of the Department of Veterans Affairs.

Service pension

This is an income-tested pension similar to the Aged and Invalid Pension provided by the Department of Social Security. It is paid to Australian veterans who have served in a theatre of war.

Supplementary assistance may be paid if you rent or board. Fringe benefits such as medical/hospital care, pharmaceutical expenses and telephone concessions are available. Applications may be made to the Department of Veterans Affairs.

Special provisions exist for veterans suffering from cancer or TB. Even if such conditions are not seen to be war-related, the veterans affected are still entitled to receive free treatment and services.

For locations of Veterans Affairs departments in other States and Territories, please see Chapter 9.

Transport benefits

■ Mobility Allowance

This is administered by the Department of Social Security. Contact your local office, which is listed in your telephone directory under the 'Commonwealth Government' section. The Allowance is a fortnightly payment to assist disabled people with transport expenses. To be eligible for benefits, individuals should:

- be unable, due to a disability, to use public transport without substantial assistance
- be at least sixteen years of age
- be employed or in vocational training for at least eight hours per week, and not have received sales tax exemption on a motor vehicle within the last two years as a result of their disabilities
- not be in receipt of a Training Allowance from the Commonwealth Rehabilitation Service

For sales tax exemption, see Chapter 14.

■ Isolated Patient Travel and Accommodation Assistance Scheme (IPTAAS) in New South Wales

This scheme is administered by the New South Wales Department of Health.

> Head office:
> IPTAAS
> 73 Miller Street
> NORTH SYDNEY NSW 2060
> Tel.: (02) 391 9491

This scheme provides financial help to people in rural areas who have to travel more than 200 kilometres from their homes in order to obtain specialist medical treatment or services. The Scheme may allow for some reimbursement of travel and accommodation costs.

An essential part of the scheme is that a medical practitioner should refer you for treatment to the nearest suitable specialist. The referring doctor is required to complete Section A of the IPTAAS application form.

Application forms are obtainable at the Regional Offices of the Department of Health or at the Social Work Department of any hospital.

ℹ️ PTAAS in other States and Territories

Queensland

Details of the Patient Transit Scheme are available from your local public hospital.

South Australia

Patient Assistance Transport Scheme
c/- SA Health Commission
11 Hindmarsh Square
ADELAIDE SA 5000
Tel.: (08) 226 7000

Victoria

Victorian Patient Travel Assistance Scheme
(VPTAS)
Tel.: (03) 616 7334 or (008) 13 3345 (toll free)

Western Australia

For application to the Patients Assistance Travel Scheme (PATS), forms are available from your local hospital, or from your GP if you live in a rural area.

In other States and Territories, contact your local hospital or GP for details of any applicable travel assistance schemes.

Accommodation

■ Rental assistance by the Department of Social Security

Persons receiving a Social Security benefit/pension can apply for rental assistance. For people who do not have children, there is a 26-week wait for rental assistance. For people who do, there is no waiting period.

The amount of assistance you receive is dependent on the amount of rent you pay per fortnight. It may also be adjusted if you have one or more children living at home with you.

■ Assistance by the Department of Housing

This department can also assist you with rent relief. In order to be eligible for this, you must have approval for Priority Housing with the Department. If suitable Department of Housing accommodation has not been found after 28 days of Priority Housing approval, you are entitled to receive subsidised rental assistance from the Department of Housing.

However, you must be prepared to forfeit your rental accommodation when suitable Department of Housing accommodation becomes available.

Depending on your circumstances, the Department of Housing can also help you pay a proportion of your bond and rent arrears.

ℹ️ Additional benefits available

■ New South Wales

There are a number of benefits paid to disabled people and/or their families. Here are some of them.

Carer's benefits

These are paid in relation to the care an individual requires from another person.

Domiciliary nursing care benefits

These are administered by:
Department of Health, Housing & Community
Services

4th Floor
120 Sussex Street
SYDNEY NSW 2000
Tel.: (02) 225 3555

This is a benefit applicable to carers of people who need full-time nursing at home. The benefit is paid on the condition that a nursing sister is calling at regular intervals and that the carer is not employed in the workforce. The benefit is not means tested.

Applications are available through Community Nursing Services, hospitals and general practitioners, and should be sent to the Department of Health.

■ Other States and Territories

Contact the head office of the Department of Health, Housing and Community Services listed in the 'Commonwealth Government' section of the *White Pages.*

■ Attendants Allowance

This is administered by the Department of Veterans Affairs. The head office address is:

300 Elizabeth Street
SYDNEY NSW 2000
Tel.: (02) 213 7777

This is an allowance for an attendant, payable to a veteran who has a disability as a result of war service. The amount of the benefit is related to the degree of disability. Applications and further information can be obtained through the Department of Veterans Affairs.

Financial advice

A number of organisations offer expertise in the area of financial counselling. These include:

Credit Line
53 Regent Street
Railway Square
SYDNEY NSW 2000
Tel.: (02) 394 7422

This scheme is a counselling service to help people with financial difficulties. It aims to assist people by giving practical advice on how to manage finances. This may include budgeting advice, negotiations in situations between people and their creditors, and education in money management. Advice is given over the telephone and by personal interview.

> Welfare Rights Centre
> 4th Floor
> 245 Castlereagh Street
> SYDNEY NSW 2000
> Tel.: (02) 267 5077

This service assists people with problems related to social security by supplying information and advice. The service assists people with problems related to the appeals process, and clarifies and reforms unfair laws and practices related to social security matters. The Centre is not meant to handle routine problems that may easily be clarified with the office concerned.

ℹ️ Legal aid centres

Many legal aid centres also have solicitors who specialise in helping people with financial problems. Here are some examples.

New South Wales

> Consumer Credit Legal Centre
> 13 Meagher Street
> CHIPPENDALE NSW 2008
> Tel.: (02) 698 9448

> Redfern Legal Aid Centre
> 71–73 Pitt Street
> REDFERN NSW 2016
> Tel.: (02) 698 7277

Queensland

> Financial Counselling Service
> 60 Barwick Street
> FORTITUDE VALLEY QLD 4006
> Tel.: 257 1957

South Australia

> Department for Family and Community Services
> Citicentre
> 11 Hindmarsh Square
> ADELAIDE SA 5000
> Tel.: (08) 226 7000

Victoria

Citizens Advice Bureau or local councils, as listed in the telephone directory.

Western Australia

> Creditcare
> 95 William Street
> PERTH WA 6000

Other States and Territories

In Tasmania, the Australian Capital Territory and Northern Territory, contact the social work department at your local hospital.

In other areas, legal aid offices are listed in the local *White Pages* and *Yellow Pages*.

CHAPTER 11

Compensation for personal injury

Many people become disabled as a result of an accident. When this happens, the question often arises: 'Can I claim compensation?' The answer to this is to be found in knowing your legal rights and being aware of the various schemes through which our State provides compensation.

To help you, we have outlined the present arrangements for compensation in New South Wales. This outline is meant only as a guideline, to assist you with recognising whether or not you have a claim.

To be sure about your legal standing, it is best to contact a solicitor skilled in the area of compensation law. The solicitor will be able to act on your behalf, establish your entitlements and ensure that you are properly compensated under the legal processes of the State for any losses you sustain.

Compensation schemes that provide for personal injury

- Common-law negligence actions
- Third party personal injury compensation
- WorkCover
- Sporting Injuries Insurance Scheme
- Victims Compensation Scheme

Common-law negligence actions

What is common-law action? Any person who can prove that his or her injuries were caused by the fault or negligence of another person may be able to claim compensation by suing that person in a court of law. An **action** is a legal proceeding in which a person demands or enforces his or her rights in a court of justice.

■ Making a claim

In order to establish a claim for common-law compensation you will have to take court action. In this process, the injured person (commonly named the **plaintiff**) will seek to show that another party (commonly named the **defendant**) caused his or her injuries and therefore should provide compensation (damages) to compensate for the injury. To succeed in such a claim, the injured person must show:

- that the defendant had a duty to take reasonable care for the safety of the plaintiff. This duty requires the defendant to take precautions so as to minimise the danger that a member of the public may be subject to as a result of the defendant's action
- that the defendant breached the above duty— that is, that he or she was in some way negligent
- that, as a result of his or her failure to care, the injured person suffered loss or damage

Once this relationship has been established, the injured person may seek to claim compensation for the losses or damages incurred.

Judgment about who is at fault is often complicated, and great care is needed to take all factors into account. Often situations arise where the person has contributed to his or her injuries by his or her own actions. This is called **contributory negligence**. In this case, the Court decides on the degree of negligence and adjusts the amount of compensation payable.

The common-law system therefore leaves many people without any claim for compensation.

■ How is this compensation paid?

Compensation takes the form of a lump sum award of 'damages', assessed on a once-and-for-all basis. The lump sum award covers both past and future losses and cannot be varied. There are two categories of compensation:

- **Special damages**: usually included in this area are all the hospital, medical, ambulance, rehabilitation and associated expenses directly resulting from the accident and also the calculation of loss of wages of the injured party.
- **General damages**: an injured person is also entitled to be compensated by way of a lump sum for the injuries, disabilities and loss of quality of

life suffered by him or her as a result of the accident. Taken into account in this amount are the types of injuries sustained by the individual, the period of hospitalisation, the pain and suffering the injured party has had to bear and any continuing disabilities experienced by the injured party.

■ Can I always be assured of compensation?

While proof of fault is essential in establishing a compensation claim in terms of the common law, it does not of itself ensure that the injured person will be able to obtain damages. If the party you are suing has no money or insurance cover, then there will be little advantage in pressing a claim. There is no universal scheme to protect people in this situation.

An exception to this is in the area of motor accidents. Here, the New South Wales government has tried to ensure that when people are injured by other road users, there will be enough money to ensure adequate common-law compensation.

Third party personal injury compensation

The Motor Accidents Scheme commenced on 1 July 1989, replacing the previous transport accident compensation scheme, Transcover. The Act covers people involved in motor accidents, and allows a claim to be made for damages or compensation in the event of the death of or injury to a person as a result of a motor accident.

It is compulsory for owners of motor vehicles in New South Wales to have third party insurance, which is taken out automatically at the time of registering the vehicle. For the first two years of operation of the scheme, the Roads and Traffic Authority had allocated insurance cover to one of 13 insurance companies. Since July 1991, vehicle owners have been able to choose their own third party insurers, and must take out the insurance before registering their vehicles.

As the scheme is fault based, insurers provide compensation only where the driver or owner of an insured vehicle is at fault or liable for injuries suffered by another arising from the use of that vehicle.

If the other driver who is at fault cannot be identified or is uninsured, claims are made against a Nominal Defendant, through the Motor Accidents Authority. The Nominal Defendant is funded by the insurance companies involved in the third party scheme.

■ The Motor Accidents Authority

The Motor Accidents Authority is an independent statutory body funded by a levy on third party premiums. Its Board of Directors includes those representing road users, accident victims, lawyers, doctors, insurers and the government.

The main functions of the Authority include:

- monitoring the operation of the Third Party Insurance Scheme
- monitoring and licensing insurance companies providing cover under the scheme
- funding initiatives for the prevention and minimisation of road accident injuries
- conducting research on motor accidents, compensation claims, damages paid to accident victims and court proceedings
- publicising and disseminating information in relation to the scheme
- monitoring the handling of claims under the old Third Party scheme by the GIO
- advising the government on the operation of the scheme and the need for further changes to ensure it provides reasonable compensation to accident victims at a cost the community can afford

■ How to make a third party personal injury compensation claim

There are several steps to follow when making a claim. First of all, you must report the accident to the police, and you must do this within *28 days* of the date of the accident.

If, because of injuries received in the accident, you are unable to make a report within the first 28 days, you may make a report within 28 days after the date by which you may reasonably have been expected to do so. Otherwise you must satisfy the court that sufficient cause existed to justify the delay in making a report.

The next step is to give a notice of claim to the driver of the other vehicle and to that vehicle's insurer. This must happen within *six months* of the accident happening.

It is generally advisable to engage a solicitor when giving notice of a claim, although it is not strictly necessary. To make a claim yourself you need to know details of the accident, vehicles involved and witnesses, if any.

If you are unsure of the compulsory Third Party insurer of the other vehicle, you should contact the Motor Accidents Authority:

Tel.: (02) 252 4677 or (008) 46 3940

or the Road Traffic Authority:

Tel.: (02) 662 5000

with the registration number of the vehicle at fault, and the authority will tell you who the insurer is.

If several vehicles are involved, you should send your claim to the insurer of the vehicle you consider to be most at fault. Claim forms are available from the insurers, the Motor Accidents Authority, or your solicitor.

A claim is not considered to have been made until the insurer has received a *completed* claim form. This means you must provide details on every section of the form. Until insurers receive a completed claim form they are not obliged to assess your claim.

On the claim form you must provide details about yourself, the accident, your injuries and treatment, any details regarding loss of earnings, a medical certificate, completed by your doctor, and a Certificate of Earnings, completed by your employer.

You may also engage a solicitor to assist with your claim. The solicitor can:

- advise whether you should seek damages following a motor vehicle accident
- collect all the information necessary for making the claim
- arrange for witnesses to testify on your behalf
- negotiate with the insurer
- advise you of any offer of settlement
- prepare and file a statement of claim in court, if necessary
- brief a barrister who will represent you in court, if necessary
- arrange for payment of accounts from any settlement or damages awarded

◼ After the claim has been lodged

Once your claim has been given to the insurer of the driver at fault, it is the duty of the insurer to try to resolve the claim as quickly as possible. It is *your* duty to co-operate with the third party insurer, and to respond to any reasonable requests to:

- provide a photograph of yourself and/or other proof of identity
- undergo medical examinations and/or other assessments

You are also expected to take all *reasonable* steps to reduce the impact of your injuries by participating in ongoing rehabilitation or undergoing medical treatment or pursuing alternative employment opportunities.

◼ What happens when the third party insurer admits liability?

Once liability has been admitted (either wholly or in part), it is the duty of the insurer to pay for hospital, medical, pharmaceutical, equipment and rehabilitation expenses as incurred.

Six months after the claim was first made, you are entitled to commence court proceedings against the other person. You will seek, in the settlement, compensation for past, present and future expenses arising from your motor vehicle accident and injury.

The third party insurer may make an offer of settlement to you prior to your claim going to court. If you and the insurer agree on an amount of compensation, the claim need not go to court at all.

Your solicitor should advise you whether the offer is a fair one. If you agree to settlement terms, you will have to sign a deed of release in which you agree to make no further claims in connection with the accident.

If your claim is determined by the Court, you will be compensated for hospital, medical, pharmaceutical and rehabilitation expenses incurred to date, as well as

for future expenses of this type. You will also be compensated for any loss of earnings, past and future. On top of this you may be paid general damages for pain and suffering, loss of amenities, disfigurement and loss of expectation of life, up to a maximum of $192 600.

Generally compensation is paid in a lump sum, but the Court may allow a 'structured settlement' for people suffering serious injury. In these cases future hospital and medical costs are paid as they are incurred, to protect people from rising medical costs.

◼ What happens if the insurer does not admit liability?

If, after you have made a claim to the other party's insurer, the following occurs:

- the insurer *denies all liability* in respect of the claim, or
- the insurer admits *partial liability* but you are unhappy with the extent to which liability is admitted,

then you are entitled to commence court proceedings immediately.

◼ What happens if I was partly at fault?

If you were partly at fault for the accident, your compensation may be reduced by an amount which the Court thinks just and equitable in the circumstances of the case.

Here are some of the cases where your compensation may be reduced and a finding of contributory negligence made against you:

- if you were partly responsible for the accident
- if, at the time of the accident, you had in your blood more than the prescribed amount of alcohol
- if you were a passenger and the driver's ability to drive the motor vehicle was impaired as a result of consumption of a drug or alcohol, and you were aware of that impairment, or should have been aware
- if you were not wearing a seat belt
- if you were not wearing a protective helmet while riding a motorcycle

◼ Benefits—rehabilitation

Once an insurer has admitted liability under a third party policy, it is obliged to provide for the rehabilitation of an injured person, and to ensure that rehabilitation services are provided as soon as possible after the motor accident. Rehabilitation means, for the injured person, the process of restoring or attempting to restore that person to the maximum level of function of which he or she is capable, or that he or she wishes to achieve.

Rehabilitation services may include:

- medical services
- social services
- educational services
- vocational services

These services may also include placement in employment, and social rehabilitation, such as family and leisure counselling and training for independent living.

The insurer may also be liable for meeting the necessary and reasonable costs and expenses of travel and accommodation incurred by the injured person as a result of obtaining rehabilitation services.

In the final assessment of damages or settlement of a claim, the extent to which the injured person undertook rehabilitation or underwent medical treatment will be taken into account. The Court will consider the extent to which the person participated in a rehabilitation program, and the onus lies with the injured person to show that he or she has participated in a program, and taken steps to mitigate or reduce damages.

■ Benefits—economic loss

The term 'economic loss' refers to:

- the loss or impairment of earning capacity, or
- the loss of expectation of financial support, or
- the liability of incurring expenditure in the future as a result of a motor vehicle accident.

The last category includes past and future medical and rehabilitation expenses, as well as certain home care services relating to nursing and attendant care.

When damages are awarded to a person who has suffered either severe permanent disability or long-term disability, the court may include an amount to cover both past and future economic loss, and may pay these damages as a structured settlement. The injured person may request a structured settlement for damages for the impairment of earning capacity, or the court may order a structured settlement if it considers there are good reasons to do so and the insurer consents to this.

If economic loss is awarded as a lump sum, it will be discounted by a small percentage rate. This is because the injured person may earn investment income on the amount awarded, so the court must estimate a sum of money that will yield the future economic loss through that investment.

The court may also reduce the amount of economic loss of an injured person if he or she is entitled to compensation under the *Victims Compensation Act* 1987.

■ Benefits—non-economic loss

Damages may be awarded to an injured person for non-economic loss if the person's ability to lead a normal life is significantly impaired by the injury. Non-economic loss means:

- pain and suffering,
- loss of amenities of life,
- loss of expectation of life or
- disfigurement.

The amount of damages awarded depends upon the severity of the non-economic loss. The maximum amount which may be awarded in the most severe case is $192 600.

If non-economic loss is assessed as $16 050 or less, the court will award no damages for non-economic loss. Between $16 050 and $42 800, the court will reduce the amount according to a specific formula.

The maximum amount of $192 600 is indexed to changes in the average weekly total earnings of adults in New South Wales working full time, estimated by the Australian Statistician.

Benefits in States and Territories other than New South Wales

For information regarding compensation for personal injury in motor vehicle accidents in your State or Territory, contact the following.

Victoria

Transport Accident Commission
Tel.: (03) 664 6666

Queensland

QAN Society
179 Anne Street
BRISBANE QLD 4000

South Australia

State Government Insurance Commission
211 Victoria Square
ADELAIDE SA 5000
Tel.: (08) 233 1111

Western Australia

State Government Insurance Commission
225 Adelaide Terrace
PERTH WA 6000

In other States and Territories, contact your solicitor for information.

WorkCover

This is a general guide to workers' compensation and related matters in New South Wales and does not claim to be exhaustive. You should consult your legal adviser in relation to specific rights or responsibilities. WorkCover is the name for the occupational health, safety, rehabilitation and compensation scheme in New South Wales. It is administered by the WorkCover Authority. The main objectives of the WorkCover scheme are to:

- improve health and safety standards at workplaces in New South Wales
- assist the worker with returning to productive work where an injury has occurred
- adequately and efficiently compensate injured workers

■ General provisions

What is workers' compensation?

Workers' compensation is basically a no-fault system providing financial benefits and other assistance to injured workers and their dependants. These are available to workers or the dependants of workers who suffer injury or disease associated with their employment which results in:

- death or incapacity for work
- permanent loss or impairment of part of the body or a faculty
- medical or hospital treatment
- the need for rehabilitation

Who can claim workers' compensation benefits?

A person who is a worker or someone deemed a worker under the *Workers' Compensation Act* may claim benefits.

Generally, a worker is someone who receives wages or commission, regardless of the number of hours worked each week, and the definition includes workers who work away from the employer's premises. Persons engaged in New South Wales to work outside the State are entitled to compensation under the law of New South Wales if they are injured.

The *Workers' Compensation Act* recognises certain other persons as workers. These include:

- a person who enters into a contract to perform work, valued in excess of $10.00, that is not part of or connected with any regular trade or business of his or her own, and performs a task without employing others or subcontracting the task
- a person who contracts to do certain kinds of rural work, including clearing land and felling timber, constructing or demolishing fences or yards, and cutting or transporting sugar cane
- salespersons who receive commission, unless it is paid in relation to a trade or business regularly carried out by the salesperson or his or her firm
- mine employees and mines rescue personnel
- jockeys and certain harness racing drivers
- drivers of hire vehicles or hire vessels
- most casual or part-time workers
- persons attending a prearranged place for pick-up
- boxers, wrestlers and the referees of their matches and entertainers in contests or performances that are held in registered clubs or where an admission fee is charged

Even if an employer has told a person that he or she is not eligible for workers compensation cover, or has required the person to sign a statement agreeing that he or she is not a worker (but perhaps a 'contractor'), that person may still be considered a worker under the law on workers compensation. There is a large body of case law on this issue, and if you are in doubt legal assistance should be sought.

Where the worker has died as a result of injury or disease associated with employment, a person totally or partially dependent upon that worker may claim benefits. If there are no dependants, reasonable funeral costs, up to a certain amount, are payable.

Who are dependants?

A dependant is a person who is either totally or partially dependent on the worker for financial support, and who falls into the following classes:

- a member of the worker's family
- a person for whom the worker stands in place of a natural parent
- a person who stands in place of a natural parent to the worker
- the divorced husband or wife of the worker who is entitled to maintenance from that worker
- a person who is not legally married to the worker but lives with the worker as the worker's husband or wife on a permanent and genuine domestic basis

Benefits for dependants

These may be paid:

- to the worker, on behalf of the dependants
- to another person, who may or may not be a dependant—for example, a surviving spouse, on behalf of children
- into a trust fund administered by the Work-Cover Authority, which then pays benefits to the dependant in a way acceptable to both the dependant and the Authority

Entitlement to benefits

A worker is entitled to benefits if:

- he or she has suffered an injury that is work-related
- he or she is suffering from an injury or disease and his or her work has contributed to the aggravation or deterioration of the condition
- the injury occurred during a work-related journey
- the injury occurred on a journey between place of abode and work, and the worker was not at fault in any way
- the injury occurred while the worker was temporarily absent from the workplace during any ordinary recess or authorised absence
- the injury has resulted in at least one of the following:
  —total or partial incapacity to perform work
  —the need for medical, hospital or rehabilitative treatment
  —the permanent, total or partial loss of the use of certain specified limbs or senses, severe facial or bodily disfigurement, loss of sexual

organs, permanent brain damage or permanent impairment of the back, neck or pelvis

Non-entitlement to benefits

A worker is not entitled to benefits if:

- he or she has deliberately injured himself/herself
- the injury is a result of his or her serious and wilful misconduct, unless death or serious and permanent disablement occurs
- the injury occurred during a journey between the worker's place of abode and the workplace, and the worker was at fault in any way

■ How to make a claim for workers' compensation benefits

Tell the employer of any injury

The employer should be told about any injury or disease as soon as possible after its occurrence. The worker must tell the employer the following:

- his or her name and address
- details of the apparent cause of the injury or disease
- the date when it happened or when the worker became aware of it

This information may be given verbally or in writing. Failure to tell the employer or make a claim for compensation within six months of the injury or disease may delay payment of benefits or prejudice the claim. This is because delays make it difficult to establish whether the injury is work-related.

Ask the employer for a claim form

The employer should supply a claim form on request. If the employer does not have one, it may be obtained from the insurer. The employer must provide the name of the insurer on request. A worker who is having difficulty obtaining a claim form should contact WorkCover Authority Advisory Services.

Obtain a doctor's certificate

If a worker suffers a work-related injury or disease that needs medical attention and time off work is required, claims for compensation must be accompanied by a WorkCover Medical Certificate.

When seeking a WorkCover Medical Certificate, the worker may ask the doctor to comment on the certificate on the apparent cause of the injury. The certificate should also specify the estimated period in which the worker will be unfit for work. If the worker feels that he or she has recovered enough to attempt a partial return to work, that worker should talk with the doctor and organise an update of the WorkCover Medical Certificate. The updated certificate should provide details about any restrictions on work ability. The worker should then request suitable employment from the employer.

Complete the claim form

To obtain any benefit, the worker must give all the information required on the claim form. The information on this form must be correct to the best of the worker's knowledge.

If the worker has any difficulties with completing the form, help should be obtained from a suitable person. If necessary, someone else can fill in the form on the worker's behalf. A copy of all documents should be kept by the worker if possible. The WorkCover Advisory Service can also be contacted for assistance.

Give documents to the employer

The completed claim form, any medical certificates and any receipts for medical or pharmaceutical expenses or other treatment should be given to the employer. The employer must forward the claim form and documents to the insurance company within seven days, and the claim will then be processed by the insurance company.

If the worker has reason to believe that the employer may not forward the claim to the insurance company within seven days, it may be sent or delivered directly to the employer's insurance company. The WorkCover Authority Advisory Services should be contacted if the employer is being unco-operative.

If the worker's employment is terminated after the initial claim, any further medical certificates and other papers should be sent directly to the insurance company by the worker.

Additional medical certificates

The worker should forward to the employer fresh medical certificates if he or she is unable to return to work after the expiry of the first certificate. The doctor's standard medical certificate may be used for this purpose.

Any further receipts or accounts for medical and other treatment or pharmaceutical supplies resulting from the injury should also be sent to the employer.

When a partially incapacitated worker is making a request to his or her employer for suitable employment, a WorkCover Medical Certificate must be used. This certificate should outline the worker's work capabilities and limitations.

■ Action taken by the employer and the insurance company

When the employer receives the worker's claim form and medical certificates, he or she must forward the documents to the insurance company within seven days. If the employer is a self-insurer the claims will be dealt with by the employer's claims section.

The insurance company will then assess the claim, and must make a decision on liability within 21 days after the claim is made. This period may be extended if there are proper reasons for more time being required.

The insurer may ask the worker to attend medical examinations. These examinations must be arranged at reasonable hours and intervals. All reasonable costs must be met by the insurer. Reasonable travelling expenses to and from the examination may be claimed.

Procedure where the claim is accepted

If the insurance company agrees to pay the claim, the worker will receive payment from either the employer or the insurer. Weekly compensation is payable either:

- at the employer's usual times of payment of wages, or
- at fortnightly or shorter intervals.

The employer/insurer and the worker may agree on other times for payment.

The employer or insurer may pay compensation in cash, by cheque, or, if the worker agrees, by means of direct credit to a bank, building society or credit union account. The worker should make a note of the claim number if the claim is accepted and quote it, together with his or her name and the employer's name, on all documents sent to the employer or insurer.

■ Medical panels

Medical panels are convened if there is a medical dispute. The injured worker's condition and fitness for employment are then assessed by the panel. Applications for a medical panel may be made by a worker, an employer, an insurer or a solicitor. The examinations are conducted by medical practitioners, usually those who are in private practice and are appointed as referees by the Chief Judge of the Compensation Court.

■ WorkCover benefits

In addition to weekly benefits, a worker may obtain:

- a lump-sum payment for the permanent loss or impairment of a specified bodily function or limb, severe facial or bodily disfigurement and related pain and suffering
- a common-law entitlement, in the case of a serious injury caused by negligence of the employer or a fellow worker
- reimbursement for medical and hospital expenses, artificial aids and house modifications
- compensation for personal items damaged in a work-related accident, such as eyeglasses
- vocational retraining
- rehabilitation assistance
- interpreter support
- legal aid

■ Other benefits

If weekly compensation is either not available or temporarily unavailable, the worker may be entitled to benefits from other government departments:

- The Commonwealth Department of Social Security provides a number of benefits for people who are out of work due to unemployment or illness. Workers should contact the nearest office of the Department of Social Security if this applies.
- The New South Wales Department of Community Services and the New South Wales Department of Housing—Home Purchases Advisory Service also provide emergency and other assistance.

■ Rights and obligations of workers

What are the rights of a dismissed worker?

The employer must not dismiss an injured worker within six months of the injury wholly or mainly because of the injury, unless the worker is permanently unable to return to his or her previous job.

A worker who has been dismissed and who is fit for his or her former position may apply to the employer for reinstatement in that position. A standard medical certificate must be produced stating that the worker is fit to resume his or her former position.

If the employer refuses to reinstate the worker, that worker may apply to the Industrial Commission for a reinstatement order.

What can be done if a claim is rejected or delayed?

If a claim for weekly benefits is rejected, the insurer will lodge a statement of dispute with the Conciliation branch of the WorkCover Authority. A conciliation officer will consider the dispute.

If the insurer rejects a claim or stops payments, the worker may ask a conciliation officer to consider the matter.

In cases where conciliation does not succeed, the worker may take the case to the Compensation Court. This court has jurisdiction to hear all workers compensation matters. Cases are allocated to either a Judge or a Commissioner, depending on the complexity of the matter. Application may be made for a review of a Commissioner's decision by a Judge of the Compensation Court.

There is a right of appeal from the Compensation Court.

Legal costs

When cases are taken before the Compensation Court, legal charges and costs will be involved. Where workers win their cases, their costs will normally be paid. Workers who do not win their cases will have to pay some of their own costs. Workers involved in claims that are 'frivolous' or 'vexatious', fraudulent or made without proper justification may be ordered to pay the other parties' costs.

Medical examination

The worker must attend medical examinations arranged by the insurer or at the direction of the WorkCover Authority, the Compensation Court, or a conciliation officer. Failure to attend without a reasonable excuse may result in suspension of the worker's right to compensation.

A worker who is required to attend a medical examination before a medical panel is entitled to recover from the employer:

- the amount of any wages lost
- the cost of fares
- maintenance costs
- travelling expenses

The worker cannot recover these costs if he or she made the application for a medical panel examination and the Compensation Court finds the application was unreasonable and unnecessary.

Penalty for false claims

A person who knowingly makes a false or misleading statement in a claim is guilty of an offence under the Act and is subject to a maximum penalty of $5000 and/or imprisonment for 12 months.

Notification of return to work

A worker who is in receipt of weekly compensation payments must immediately notify the person making the payments if:

- he or she commences employment elsewhere or is in his or her own business, or
- if there is any change in employment that affects his or her earnings.

The maximum penalty for failing to do this is $2000.

Refund of weekly payments

The Court may order a worker to refund money to which he or she is not entitled because of a return to work or an increase in earnings. This could happen if a worker:

- is no longer entitled to weekly compensation and has continued to receive it, or
- has received a higher weekly amount of compensation than he or she is entitled to receive.

Rehabilitation training

A worker's co-operation in any rehabilitation program is an important factor in the successful return to suitable employment.

If an employer does not provide suitable employment as requested by a partially incapacitated worker, the worker may undertake rehabilitation training or seek suitable employment elsewhere. In these circumstances additional weekly compensation entitlements may be available.

If the worker unreasonably refuses an offer of suitable employment or rehabilitation training, or refuses to have an assessment made of employment prospects, these additional payments may not be available.

Occupational health and safety

A worker must take reasonable care in relation to the health and safety of others and co-operate with the employer's efforts to comply with occupational health and safety requirements. This includes participating in regular health and safety meetings and reporting any potential hazards in the workplace.

Weekly payments on return to work

Although a partially incapacitated person may return to work, doing so may mean he or she will earn less than before the injury. The reasons could be that:

- he or she is working part-time,
- he or she is working full time, but is unable to do overtime or work on more highly paid shifts as was possible before the injury, and/or
- he or she is working on appropriate duties as part of the workplace rehabilitation program.

Workers compensation benefits may be paid to make up the difference between the worker's current reduced earnings and pre-injury earnings.

Weekly payments while undergoing rehabilitation

A partially incapacitated worker may undertake or complete rehabilitation even though the employer is unable or unwilling to provide 'suitable employment'. Where the employer fails to provide suitable employment as requested by a partially incapacitated worker, increased benefits may be paid for a maximum period of 52 weeks.

The benefit is available only if it is reasonably necessary for the worker to undergo rehabilitation in order to secure employment. The benefit is not available if the employer has offered suitable employment.

Further information for workers

Uninsured Liability and Indemnity Scheme

Workers can claim against this scheme if:

- they are unable to identify their employers, after careful searching, or
- the employer does not have a workers' compensation insurance policy and is unable or unwilling to meet their claims.

Alternatives to workers' compensation

In some cases, a worker may be able to institute legal action against other parties. This could be possible if it appears that the injury was caused by the negligence or breach of statutory duty of a third party who is not:

- the employer,
- a fellow employee, or
- someone else for whom the employer may be liable.

Third party insurance

If the injury arose out of a motor vehicle accident, the worker may be able to claim under the Compulsory Third Party Insurance Scheme administered by the Motor Accidents Authority.

Worker's right to common-law remedies

A seriously injured worker should seek legal advice before deciding whether to sue the employer or to accept any lump-sum workers compensation.

Taxation of compensation benefits

Taxation laws change from time to time. Therefore the worker should always check with a solicitor, accountant or the Commonwealth Taxation Office as to which benefits are taxable.

Sick pay and holiday pay

If the worker has received sick pay for any period in which he or she is also entitled to weekly compensation, the sick leave will be recredited when payments commence. The employer will be reimbursed by the insurer for the sick leave already paid, from the weekly compensation payable for that period.

If the worker has received holiday pay or long-service leave for any period in which he or she is entitled to weekly compensation, the amount of weekly compensation will not be reduced. If a public holiday or award holiday falls within the period of certified incapacity, in accordance with the Act this day is deemed to be payable by way of compensation benefits.

Therefore, the employer will not be reimbursed for the leave payments, and the worker will receive the full amount of weekly compensation payments payable for the period off work.

Interpreters

Interpreters may be arranged for:

- the discussion of approved rehabilitation programs
- medical examinations arranged by the insurer
- legal conferences and hearings before the Compensation Court or conciliation officers
- consultation with the medical panel

Where an employer or insurer has asked the worker to be medically examined and an interpreter is required, the insurer is responsible for arranging an interpreter and paying for such services.

The Telephone Interpreter Service of the Department of Immigration, Local Government and Ethnic Affairs provides free telephone interpreting and face-to-face interpreting to individuals, doctors, non-government non-profit organisations and community groups. Cost recovery provisions apply for services to other organisations.

The Ethnic Affairs Commission of New South Wales provides an interpreting and translating service. These services are provided on a fee-for-service basis.

Some of the WorkCover Authority publications are available in a number of community languages.

For further information, that is, if you have any general or any specific inquiries regarding workers compensation, contact your solicitor, personnel officer, union or the WorkCover Authority's Advisory Section at the following address:

400 Kent Street
SYDNEY NSW 2000
Tel.: (02) 370 5000

Please note: This information is a general guide to workers compensation and related matters in New South Wales, and does not claim to be exhaustive. Legislation changes regularly, and you should consult your legal advisor in relation to specific rights or responsibilities.

WorkCover authorities in States and Territories other than New South Wales

Western Australia

Workers Compensation Rehabilitation
Commission
2 Bedbrook Place
SHENTON PARK WA 6008

Queensland

Workers Compensation Board
280 Adelaide Street
BRISBANE QLD 4000

Victoria

Work Care
Tel.: (03) 603 1444

South Australia

WorkCover Compensation
100 Waymouth Street
ADELAIDE SA 5000
Tel.: (08) 233 2222

For other States and Territories, contact your solicitor for information.

New South Wales Sporting Injuries Insurance Scheme

The Sporting Injuries Insurance Scheme was created to provide some compensation to people who are seriously injured while participating in a sporting activity.

The scheme provides personal accident and injury cover for members of those sporting organisations that have elected to join it. These members may be registered players, competitors or contestants, or other participants, such as referees, umpires, coaches, managers, judges and marshals.

A lump-sum benefit is paid to any person who is injured while participating in an authorised activity or sporting event and who has suffered a permanent disability of a certain kind. The amount of the payment will vary depending on the severity of the injury. Should the injury result in death, a benefit may be paid to the legal personal representative of the deceased.

■ What sporting activities are covered?

These are:

- all normal competition matches, sporting events and fixtures
- exhibition and trial events
- organised and supervised practice and training sessions

■ How to make a claim

Claims are usually made through the sporting organisation, and should be submitted to the Sporting Injuries Committee. Remember that the claim must be lodged with the Committee within one year of the date of injury.

■ The Supplementary Sporting Injuries Scheme in New South Wales

This scheme provides compensation similar to that provided by the main scheme, compensating those injured while participating in school sport or engaged in specific programs conducted by the Department of Sport, Recreation and Racing. It is a non-contributory scheme that is totally funded by the New South Wales government.

■ Further information

Committee staff are on hand to assist with any inquiries, and can be contacted at the following address:

The Sporting Injuries Committee
Level One
115 Pitt Street
SYDNEY NSW 2000
Tel.: (02) 232 6500
Fax: (02) 221 1267

■ Compensation in States and Territories other than New South Wales

Contact your solicitor to clarify what your rights and entitlements may be.

The New South Wales Victims Compensation Scheme

This scheme was established by the New South Wales Task Force on Services for Victims of Crime in 1987. It is designed to provide a sensitive, accessible and speedy mechanism for financially compensating victims of violent crime.

■ Can I claim compensation under the scheme?

You are eligible to claim compensation if:

- you were the victim of an act of violence and are injured as a result
- you are injured as a result of witnessing an act of violence or becoming aware of it in some other way
- you are the husband or wife or de facto husband or wife, parent or child of a person killed as the result of an act of violence
- you are injured in the course of law enforcement while trying to:
  - —prevent someone from committing an offence,
  - —arrest someone who is committing an offence, or
  - —help or rescue someone against whom an offence is being committed.

■ How much can I claim?

The maximum award that can be granted is $50 000. Of this amount, up to $40 000 can be awarded for personal injuries and up to $1000 for the loss of personal effects. There is no restriction on the amount that can be awarded for expenses, as long as the total award does not exceed $50 000. (These amounts may change over time.)

■ May a child claim?

Yes, a child may claim: if a child is the victim of an act of violence, an application may be made by a relative or other suitable person on that child's behalf. Any award that is made will be held in trust (usually by the Public Trustee) and managed on behalf of the child until he or she is 18 years of age.

■ What types of injuries can I claim for?

The Victims Compensation Scheme is designed to provide compensation for bodily harm, nervous shock, mental illness or disorder, or pregnancy, resulting from acts of violence.

Compensation is available under the scheme for:

- pain and suffering
- loss of enjoyment of life
- loss of earnings
- medical expenses
- loss of personal effects
- other incidental expenses

In the case of an injury causing death, funeral expenses, grief and loss of support can also be claimed.

If you wish to make a claim, you should keep a record of all expenses incurred as a result of the injury, including details of any medical treatment you have had. Even if you receive money under the scheme, you can still take action for damages through the courts. Your solicitor or a Chamber Magistrate will be able to advise you on whether this is appropriate in your case.

■ What types of claims are *not* covered by the scheme?

In some circumstances an award of compensation may not be made. This includes cases where:

- a victim does not report the offence to the

police within a reasonable time (unless it can be established that the delay was justified)

- a victim does not help the police in their inquiries regarding the arrest or prosecution of an accused person
- it cannot be proved that an act of violence occurred
- the amount of compensation is less than $200
- the claim arises from a crime against property
- the claim arises from injuries caused by a motor vehicle and the victim is entitled to claim Compulsory Third Party Insurance benefits
- the claim is for expenses and losses that can be recovered from another source—for example, medical expenses that can be recovered from Medicare, or lost income that can be recovered under WorkCover

■ Is my behaviour at the time of the incident relevant?

Yes, it is. An award may be reduced or refused if the Tribunal considers that the victim's behaviour contributed to his or her injury or death.

■ When should I make a claim?

You should make a claim to the Victims Compensation Tribunal within two years of the date of the act of violence, but in most cases it is best to make the claim as soon as possible after the incident.

If your claim is more than two years old, the Tribunal may still allow you to make a claim, but you will need to make a special application for this. The Victims Compensation Tribunal staff will explain to you how to make a special application.

You do not have to lay charges against the person who is accused of committing the crime before you make your claim. It is also possible for your claim to be finalised before an offender is identified or dealt with by a court.

■ How do I make a claim?

Applications for an award of compensation are made to:

The Registrar
Victims Compensation Tribunal
GPO Box 6
SYDNEY NSW 2001

If you wish to make a claim, you should write to the Registrar and give details of the date, place and circumstances of the act of violence, and the name of the police officer and police station involved in the investigations. You will then be sent an application form to complete and return.

You can also lodge your application at your local courthouse, where the court staff will help you complete the application form and will then refer it to the Tribunal for you.

■ Do I have to attend a hearing?

You will normally be able to choose either to attend or to be absent from a hearing. If you would prefer the Tribunal to decide your case without a hearing, you should inform the Registrar.

■ Do I need a solicitor?

You may make the application yourself if you wish, be represented by a lawyer, or have someone else speak for you. You can take family or friends with you for support.

■ Can I get an interpreter if I have trouble speaking or understanding English?

Yes. The Tribunal Registry staff can arrange for an interpreter to accompany you to the Tribunal hearing.

■ Where will the hearing be?

Hearings are usually held at the Tribunal's premises in Sydney. The Tribunal can also sit in various locations outside Sydney as the need arises.

■ What will happen at the hearing?

Hearings are conducted before a Tribunal Member, who is also a magistrate. They take place in an informal manner and with as little legal technicality as possible.

The Tribunal Member will consider evidence of the nature and extent of the injury. This evidence will usually take the form of written reports, including doctors' assessments of the injuries suffered, and evidence of any claim for loss of income and medical, hospital and other expenses. You will also be given the opportunity to tell the Tribunal Member anything else you think might support your claim.

■ Can I be paid in advance?

Yes, you can. If you are suffering severe financial hardship, or if some other compelling circumstance exists, the Tribunal may make an interim award before your claim is finalised. This will be deducted from the final award payment.

■ Will my privacy be protected?

The Tribunal can order that hearings are closed to the public, and that material that is likely to identify the person making the claim is not published.

■ Will the offender be there?

No, the offender will not be there. The person who committed or is accused of committing the crime will not participate in the compensation hearing. He or she will not receive notice of your application, or be involved in the compensation proceedings in any way.

■ Do I have to pay costs?

An applicant is entitled to be paid his or her costs for the proceedings in accordance with a scale of costs prescribed by the rules of the Tribunal. These costs are paid over and above the amount of the compensation award. Your lawyer cannot charge you any more than the amount awarded for costs by the Tribunal.

■ Will the offender have to pay?

Yes, the offender will have to pay. If a person is convicted of the crime for which you are claiming compensation, and the Tribunal awards you a sum of money, the Tribunal can take action to recover the money from the offender. You will not have to give evidence or be involved in these proceedings.

■ Do I have a right to appeal?

If you disagree with the Tribunal's decision, you can appeal to the District Court. If you wish to appeal, you will have to lodge the appeal within two months of the date of notification of the Tribunal's decision.

■ Further information (New South Wales)

The Victims Compensation Tribunal
Level 1
Downing Centre
143–147 Liverpool Street
SYDNEY NSW 2000
Tel.: (02) 287 7154

In the remaining States and Territories, contact your solicitor to clarify what your rights and entitlements may be.

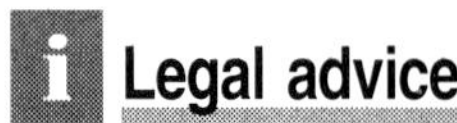 Legal advice

■ New South Wales

Concern, after an injury, about your legal situation and compensation entitlements can be an added and unnecessary stress. As mentioned above, it is best to contact a solicitor skilled in the area of compensation law in order to have your legal position and compensation entitlements clarified. Legal advice can be sought from the following organisations.

■ The Law Society of New South Wales

For free legal advice, contact:

Community Assistance Department
The Law Society
Tel.: (02) 232 2511

The Law Society can also provide a comprehensive list of solicitors and legal firms with experience in compensation law. Though very few solicitors will not ask any fee at all for an initial consultation, all should be able to advise you immediately of fee schedules or of your eligibility for legal aid. For more information, contact:

The Law Society of New South Wales
170 Phillip Street
SYDNEY NSW 2000
Tel.: (02) 220 0333

■ The Legal Aid Commission of New South Wales

The Legal Aid Commission co-ordinates the provision of free legal advice and representation throughout New South Wales. Though the Commission provides free legal advice to all, whether or not you qualify for legal representation will depend on how much money you earn and your overall financial position. If you choose to contact a private solicitor you can also make an application for legal aid through him or her.

Branch offices in Sydney and regional rural areas can be found in the 'State Government' section of the *White Pages*. In those rural areas where there is no legal aid office, the Commission pays private solicitors who specialise in its work.

Head office:
Daking House
11–23 Rawson Place
Railway Square
SYDNEY NSW 2000
Tel.: (02) 219 5711

■ Community legal centres

These centres also provide free legal advice. The Legal Aid Commission can advise you of other locations:

Tel.: (02) 219 5711

Kingsford Legal Centre
11 Rainbow Street
KINGSFORD NSW 2032
Tel.: (02) 398 6366

Redfern Legal Centre
73 Pitt Street
REDFERN NSW 2016
Tel.: (02) 698 7277

■ Aboriginal Legal Service

This service helps people of Aboriginal or Torres Strait Island descent with their legal problems. For more information, contact:

The Aboriginal Legal Service
201 Cleveland Street
REDFERN NSW 2016
Tel.: (02) 699 9277

■ WorkCover

The WorkCover Authority administers a legal aid scheme that will grant aid, in appropriate cases, to workers who cannot afford to take proceedings to the Compensation Court. Inquiries should be made to:

The WorkCover Authority
Tel.: (02) 891 0433

■ Unions

Unions should also be able to put you in contact with solicitors who can give legal advice on work-related matters.

ℹ Legal aid offices in other States and Territories

Queensland

Legal Aid Office Queensland
44 Herschel Street
BRISBANE QLD 4000

South Australia

Legal Services Commission
82–98 Wakefield Street
ADELAIDE SA 5000
Tel.: (08) 224 1222

Law Society of South Australia
124 Waymouth Street
ADELAIDE SA 5000
Tel.: (08) 231 9972

Victoria

Victorian Law Institute
Tel.: (03) 602 5000

Legal Aid Commission
Tel.: (03) 607 0234

Western Australia

Legal Aid Commission of Western Australia
105 St Georges Terrace
PERTH WA 6000

Law Society of Western Australia
33 Barrack Street
PERTH WA 6000

Sussex Street Law Centre
29 Sussex Street
VICTORIA PARK WA 6100

Residents of Tasmania, Northern Territory and Australian Capital Territory should contact the social work department at their local hospitals for further information.

ℹ Legal aid in other States and Territories

Australian Capital Territory

Tel.: (06) 243 3411

Northern Territory

Tel.: (089) 81 4799

Queensland

Tel.: (07) 238 3444

South Australia

Tel.: (08) 205 0111

Tasmania

Tel.: (002) 34 6544

Victoria

Tel.: (03) 607 0234
also contact:

Crimes Compensation Tribunal
Tel.: (03) 520 7511

Western Australia

Tel.: (09) 261 6222
also contact:

The Assessor of Criminal Injuries Compensation
105 St Georges Terrace
PERTH WA 6000

CHAPTER 12

Equipment

After you have sustained a spinal injury, you will find you will need some equipment that will enable you to live as independently as possible. The following questions frequently arise.

What equipment will I need?

This will depend largely on the level of your disability. Items may include a wheelchair (manual or power operated (electric)), cushions, a shower/commode chair (or bathseat for showering), a special bed, mattress, hoist (for lifting and transferring), and other items such as urinary gear (uridomes, leg bags, etc.).

Do I choose my own equipment?

Yes, but you should do this in consultation with other staff, such as your occupational therapist, physiotherapist and registered nurse. They can help you order the equipment that best suits your needs.

Choices are also limited by factors such as your financial situation, the availability of equipment or insurance company approval.

Do I pay for my equipment?

That depends largely on your financial situation and entitlement to compensation. There are several schemes available that offer help.

■ Schemes available in New South Wales

Program of Aids for Disabled People (PADP)

This scheme is funded by the Commonwealth Department of Health, Housing and Community Services, and is administered by hospitals throughout the city and country areas of Australia. (The scheme may be known by different names in different Australian States.)

PADP is designed to supply equipment and aids to disabled people. These aids include: wheelchairs, braces, calipers, splints, corsets and footwear; aids for incontinence, such as catheters, tubing, drainage bags and bottles; walking aids, and equipment and appliances for personal use, such as tables, beds and commode chairs.

The original intent of the scheme was to supply aids to people who require them for a disability and are ineligible to receive them under any other government-funded program, such as the programs of the Commonwealth Rehabilitation Service (the CRS), the Department of Veterans Affairs, and other State programs that provide certain aids.

In practice, the scheme has not always followed the initial guidelines. Often, individual hospitals apply their own income tests and have cut back on the range of aids and assistance they provide. It is difficult, therefore, to give a precise interpretation of the scheme and its eligibility requirements.

Most people without insurance claims use this scheme to obtain equipment while they are in a spinal unit. Once you have been discharged from the unit you must go to your nearest local hospital and make a new application for the scheme. Your local PADP will then take over the financing, ordering and repair of equipment if you meet its eligibility requirements.

ℹ Schemes available in other States and Territories

Queensland

The Home Medical Aid Scheme is available: contact your local Community Health Centre or local public hospital for details.

South Australia

Disabled Persons Equipment Scheme (DPES)
Statewide Health Services Division
Citicentre
11–13 Hindmarsh Square
ADELAIDE SA 5000
Tel.: (08) 226 6264

<u>Victoria</u>

Community Services
Tel.: (03) 412 7625

<u>Western Australia</u>

Independent Living Centre
3 Lemnos Street
SHENTON PARK WA 6008

In other States and Territories, contact your local hospital for details of applicable equipment provision schemes.

■ Other sources of funding and equipment

The Department of Veterans Affairs

Funding for equipment from Veterans Affairs is dependent on the type of benefit you receive. In New South Wales, Veterans Affairs advises that it is best to confirm your eligibility by contacting the Domiciliary Support Section at Concord Hospital. Once eligibility is established, an occupational therapist is required to do an assessment, with recommendations for equipment purchases. Applications and enquiries should be directed to:

Domiciliary Support Section
Repatriation General Hospital
CONCORD NSW 2137
Tel.: (02) 736 6016

Commonwealth Rehabilitation Service (CRS)

The CRS will provide equipment to people who are eligible for rehabilitation assistance, if their equipment needs have been identified as being part of a rehabilitation program. In some circumstances an employed disabled person may also be eligible for the provision of workplace aids if there is evidence that that person would lose his or her job without this assistance. Contact your local CRS to clarify your eligibility. Offices are listed in the *White Pages* under 'Commonwealth Department of Health, Housing and Community Services'.

Insurance companies, WorkCover

If you have a claim for compensation and liability is not in dispute, the insurance scheme may pay for your equipment prior to settlement.

■ Service clubs and trust funds

New South Wales

Service clubs, such as the Lions Club, Rotary International and Apex, may help individuals purchase particular items of equipment. Trust funds such as the following may also be able to provide assistance:

John Farragher Trust Fund
PENRITH NSW 2750
Tel.: (047) 31 5555

This is a body that financially assists people who have become disabled through sporting accidents. The Fund aims to assist people who may need a special piece of equipment or aid for their rehabilitation and future independence.

Individuals who apply must have become disabled as a result of a sporting injury. Each person is assessed by the Trust's Board, which then determines eligibility for the scheme. Letters of application should be sent to:

Foundation for the Disabled
Locked Bag 322
PENRITH NSW 2750

Other States and Territories

Contact the Social Worker at your local hospital for details.

■ Sales tax exemption

For those people who are not eligible for assistance under the above schemes, it is worth noting that you don't have to pay sales tax for certain items—it is *not* included in the price of manual and electric wheelchairs, electrically operated beds, hydraulic lifting devices and stair-climbing devices.

However, individual claims for sales tax exemptions have to be made for the following items:

- battery chargers used for recharging electric-wheelchair batteries
- goods used in the modification of motor vehicles
- motor vehicles:
  - if your disability is a result of service in the defence force and the motor vehicle is for your own use
  - if your disability permanently prevents you from using public transport
  - if the motor vehicle purchased is for your own use in travelling to and from work

For information about how to claim an exemption, contact your local tax office.

Equipment checklist

After your discharge, most of the decision making regarding your equipment will be up to you. It is important that you know your requirements and the avenues of help available. You could consider the following.

■ Know what equipment you are using and why you need it

Learn how to describe your equipment; for example, for your wheelchair, know the seat width, back height, type of castors, number of axle settings etc. You cannot reorder what you cannot name. Make a list of your equipment.

It is important also to know why you need a particular item. This will help you to appreciate its usefulness and will also aid you if you need to justify its reordering.

■ Know what equipment is available

This is not always an easy task, as there is a great range of equipment that is constantly being updated. If you need advice and help to negotiate the system, then the best move is to contact one or all of the following:

- an occupational therapist or registered nurse at the Spinal Unit or your local hospital or Community Health Centre
- the Paraquad Association of New South Wales or the Australian Quadriplegic Association

Independent Living Centres

Independent Living Centres provide information about commercially available products for people with disabilities. The centres have a wide range of equipment on display (no device is for sale), covering various aspects of daily living including bathrooms and toilets, building modifications, wheelchairs, devices for getting dressed, means of communication, devices for driving, eating and drinking, hoists and lifting equipment, kitchens, and means of recreation, transport and employment.

If you want to organise a general tour of the centres or trial specific items, it is recommended that you make an appointment. In this way you can make sure that a staff member will be available to help you.

Australian Capital Territory

24 Parkinson Street
WESTON ACT 2611
Tel.: (06) 287 1644
Fax: (06) 287 1640

New South Wales

600 Victoria Road/PO Box 706
RYDE NSW 2112
Tel.: (02) 808 2233

New Zealand

14 Erson Avenue
ROYAL OAK AUCKLAND
NEW ZEALAND
Tel.: (64) (9) 65 8067

Queensland

Ward 1
Greenslopes Hospital
GREENSLOPES QLD 4120
Tel.: (07) 394 7471
Fax: (07) 394 1013

South Australia

180 Daws Road
DAW PARK SA 5041
Tel.: (08) 276 3455
Fax: (08) 276 7417

Victoria

52 Thistlethwaite Street/PO Box 88
SOUTH MELBOURNE VIC 3205
Tel.: (03) 690 9177
Fax: (03) 696 1956

Western Australia

3 Lemnos Street
SHENTON PARK WA 6008
Tel.: (09) 382 2011
Fax: (09) 382 7351

How do I maintain my equipment?

Funding for reordering, servicing and repairing your equipment will depend on how it was initially funded.

■ PADP

Your local scheme will co-ordinate your equipment needs.

■ Veterans Affairs

The Department will continue to supply, repair and service equipment for all eligible veterans.

■ The CRS

Items provided by the CRS will only be maintained for six months after the completion of a rehabilitation program. After that time clients will be fully responsible for any repairs, maintenance, service and replacement costs.

■ Private purchases

Ongoing equipment needs and maintenance can be organised either directly through the supplier, or through an agent such as the Paraquad Association. Maintenance can also be provided by the New South Wales Society for Children and Young Adults with Physical Disabilities, which has a maintenance service for wheelchairs, hoists and other equipment.

For further information:

Tel.: (02) 890 0100

■ Know how long things will last

This will ensure that you always have an adequate and continuous supply. This is especially important to remember in relation to your urinary gear. It will also help you to decide when equipment has outlived its usefulness; this is worth knowing in relation to, for example, cushions (consult the Paraplegic and Quadriplegic Association).

■ Organisations for special equipment needs

There are some organisations that operate to help people with disabilities with particular equipment needs. One such body is Technical Aid for the Disabled (TAD).

TAD groups are non-profit organisations made up of volunteer professional engineers, technicians and tradespeople who lend their expertise to help overcome architectural and equipment problems faced by people with disabilities. It is TAD's aim to design, construct, install and maintain devices for clients where commercial equipment is not available.

Though TAD volunteers make no charge for their labour, clients are asked to cover the cost of materials where possible. TAD is also able to provide information about devices, appropriate technology, available expertise, material suppliers and industrial facilities, and produces a journal that details the latest advances in equipment for people with disabilities.

Australian Capital Territory

TAD ACT Inc.
20 Muresk Street
FARRAR ACT 2607
Tel.: (06) 286 3136
Fax: (06) 290 1470

New South Wales

227 Morrison Road / PO Box 108
RYDE NSW 2112
Tel.: (02) 808 2022

Queensland

TAD Queensland
PO Box 257
ANNERLEY QLD 4103
Tel.: (07) 397 8987
Fax: (07) 397 9020

Queensland Technical Groups are located in Bundaberg, Cairns, Gold Coast, Mackay, Rockhampton, Sunshine Coast, Toowoomba and Townsville.

South Australia

Technical Aid to the Disabled (SA) Inc.
PO Box 112
EASTWOOD SA 5063
Tel.: (08) 261 2922

Tasmania

TAS TAD
Room 107
Douglas Parker Rehabilitation Centre
31 Tower Road
NEW TOWN TAS 7008

Victoria

TAD VIC Co-operative Ltd
PO Box 88
SOUTH MELBOURNE VIC 3205
Tel.: (03) 698 5327
Fax: (03) 698 5328

Victorian branches are in Bairnsdale, Ballarat, Bendigo, Geelong and Shepparton.

Western Australia

Technical Aid to the Disabled WA
Suite 5
Westrade Centre
Newcastle & Lord Streets
PERTH WA 6000

CHAPTER 13

Support associations

There are a number of organisations that represent the needs and interests of disabled people. Some of these cater specifically for people with spinal injuries, while others hope to represent disabled people in general.

It is not possible to supply a comprehensive list here of all the current organisations. We have listed only the organisations that represent people with spinal cord injuries, and a few others that warrant particular mention.

These organisations offer a range of benefits. They can assist you with practical problems and with increasing your awareness of services and resources through their newsletters and magazines, they can provide a means of contacting people in circumstances similar to your own, and they can provide you with a voice to speak out on issues that affect you, in the hope that you can help improve services for all disabled people.

As these organisations are dependent on their membership, we would encourage you to join them and lend your support.

The Paraplegic and Quadriplegic Association of New South Wales (Paraquad)

33–35 Burlington Road
HOMEBUSH NSW 2140
Tel.: (02) 764 4166

and

57 Albert Street
WICKHAM NSW 2303
Tel.: (049) 69 6388

This association is an organisation for assisting, informing and supporting disabled people and their families, their friends and other concerned individuals. It aims to provide a wide range of services to its members in the areas of accommodation, supply of medical equipment, counselling, driver training etc.

■ Services

Supply of medical equipment

A large range of medications and products for caring for the bladder, bowel and skin is available at a discounted price to members.

Counselling

There are three full-time rehabilitation officers, each with expertise in the field of spinal injuries, offering advice, counselling and follow-up home visits to members.

Journals

Paraquad News and *Northern News* are quarterly information journals that provide information and promote discussion on issues relevant to people with spinal injuries.

Accommodation

The Association has built, and maintains, a 42 bed nursing home at:

Ferguson Lodge
LIDCOMBE NSW 2141

The Association also provides temporary accommodation at Berala in Sydney as a transitional step between being in a hospital or other dependent environment and living independently in the community. Five single units are available, as well as four two-bedroom houses and two three-bedroom houses.

Recreation

The Association provides both specialised and integrated recreation and leisure programs for members.

■ Membership

Any paraplegic or quadriplegic, or any other interested person, may become a member by contacting the Association.

The Australian Quadriplegic Association (AQA)

1 Jennifer Street
LITTLE BAY NSW 2036
Tel.: (02) 661 8855

AQA is an organisation that is concerned with the interests of quadriplegics. It aims to provide accommodation, employment, welfare counselling and assistance for disabled people. It helps to raise awareness, both at a government and public level, of the needs of disabled people, and acts as a lobby group to promote schemes that will alleviate the problems disabled people encounter.

■ Services

Employment

AQA headquarters at Little Bay offers work in marketing, finance and administration. The Workshop at Botany offers general contract work plus internal collating and marketing in its printing department.

Accommodation

The following is available:

- *Ashton House, Maroubra:* supported accommodation for 18 disabled people
- *Kimberley Lodge, Chifley:* a boarding house for eight disabled people
- *Stuart House, Maroubra:* Housing Commission accommodation for four disabled people
- *Coffs Harbour House:* transitional and respite accommodation for four disabled people
- *Dapto House, Wollongong:* transitional and respite accommodation for four disabled people

Welfare goods

These are supplied to members at a discount price.

Welfare advice and follow-up

Counselling services are available for advice and referrals for a range of positions.

Transport

This is offered to people in the Eastern Suburbs; the service runs to and from AQA for work and some recreational programs.

Recreation program

Outings are organised for each weekend.

Advocacy

AQA lobbies all areas of government and the community on matters affecting disabled people, and will act on behalf of individual members.

Publications

AQA offers two informative publications:

- *AQA News*—provided monthly to all members
- *Quad Wrangle*—a quarterly publication, for all people interested

■ Membership

This is open to any quadriplegic or other interested person.

ACROD Ltd

ACROD is a federation of organisations and individuals concerned with improving all aspects of the lifestyles of disabled people. Its aims are to improve services and legislation for Australians with disabilities, and to promote community acceptance of the right of people with disabilities to participate on an equal footing in all facets of society. Here are contact details:

33 Thesiger Court
DEAKIN ACT 2600
PO Box 60
CURTIN ACT 2605
Tel : (062) 82 4333

■ Membership

This is open to people with disabilities and those with a professional or personal interest in the rehabilitation of the disabled. Membership may be obtained by applying to the head office.

Disabled People's International (DPI) New South Wales

39 Morley Avenue
ROSEBERY NSW 2018
Tel.: (02) 552 1411

The DPI is an organisation set up to represent the opinions, ideas and needs of disabled people. It aims to act as an advisory body and lobby group to the government and the community so that disabled people can have a voice on issues that affect their lives, such as access and accommodation.

■ Services

The DPI not only provides an information, education and advocacy service for people with disabilities, but also plays an active role in identifying gaps in current services and providing information on resources, available support and the rights of disabled people.

■ Membership

This is open to anyone, and can be obtained by contacting the DPI Office.

Paraparents

This is a support group for parents who are in wheelchairs. 'Paraparents' meet regularly to share ideas about and experiences with bringing up their children. The group is organised by a 'wheelchair mum' and her husband. For further information, contact:

Paraplegic and Quadriplegic Association of NSW
Tel.: (02) 764 4166

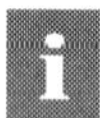 ## Other organisations

Queensland

Paraplegic & Quadriplegic Association Inc.
28 Horan Street
WEST END QLD 4101
Tel.: (07) 844 7311

South Australia

Disabled Persons International
c/- Thebarton Primary School
Rose Street
MILE END SA 5031
Tel.: (08) 234 0708

Paraplegic & Quadriplegic Association of South Australia Inc. (PQA)

Units 8 & 9
Regency Park Centre
Days Road
REGENCY PARK SA 5010
PO Box 283
KILKENNY SA 5009

Tasmania

Australian Quadriplegic Association
Tel.: (003) 27 1017

Victoria

Australian Quadriplegic Association (VIC)
70 Station Street
FAIRFIELD VIC 3078
Tel.: (03) 489 0777

Disability Resource Centre
Tel.: (03) 480 2877

Disabled Persons' Information Bureau
Tel.: (03) 412 7176

Paraquad
229 Burwood Road
HAWTHORN VIC 3121
Tel.: (03) 819 4055

Western Australia

Disability Resource Centre
189 Royal Street
EAST PERTH WA 6004

Disability Rights Service
79 Stirling Street
PERTH WA 6000

Paraquad Association
Selby Street
SHENTON PARK WA 6008

CHAPTER 14

Transportation

Freedom to get around is an essential part of being independent. Having suitable and accessible transportation helps you to achieve this goal. Public transport services are often not wheelchair-accessible, so your main options revolve around motor vehicle transportation.

Driving

Many characteristics affect a person's ability to learn or relearn how to drive. Many factors also affect the individual's ability to be transported by others. Things to be considered are:

- the type of car
- the person's position when seated in the car
- the person's level of function
- the controls available

■ The type of car

These are the requirements for enabling driving:

- automatic transmission
- power steering
- power-assisted braking
- air conditioning (necessary for quadriplegics)

These car features affect transfers:

- the opening space of the door
- whether there are bench or bucket seats (depending on the type of transfer)
- the position in which the seat can be placed
- the presence of hand holds (used by some people in their transfer)
- the individual's degree of independence, on his or her own and with a wheelchair

■ The driver's position when seated in the car

Many factors need to be considered, as with the able-bodied individual:

- the ability to reach all the available controls

- whether seating is comfortable
- whether vision zones are good (including vision necessary with mirrors)
- leg room
- skin sensitivity
- the accessibility of seat belts
- the amount of space in the car (for example, for the placement of wheelchairs)

■ The person's level of function

Many factors need to be considered here:

- physical strength, particularly shoulder movements against resistance
- the degree of controlled movement
- the degree of spasm
- the level of fatigue likely
- balance, trunk control and body-righting ability
- concentration span
- perceptual deficits
- visual problems
- lower-limb sensation
- reaction time
- the ability to manipulate controls and switches (including emergency controls, handbrake, horn, internal light)

■ The controls available

Adaptations of any sort must be made to suit the individual, but must be approved by the Department of Motor Transport Engineering Division. In certain cases the Department may wish to inspect these adaptations personally. Adaptations mean attaching steering, brake and accelerator controls to an automatic car with power steering and power-assisted brakes.

Types of hand controls

MPS Monarch Control (right-angle/push hand control)

- a push-away movement for the brake

- a pull-down movement towards the floor (at 90° angle) for the accelerator

These controls are available in kit form and can be fitted by any mechanic.

Push–pull variety

- a push-away movement for the brake
- a pull movement towards the face for acceleration

Throttle control (twist grip)

- a push-away movement for the brake
- a throttle movement—a twisting action (similar to that in motor bike control) for acceleration

Additional controls

Controls such as these may be necessary for activating systems other than the accelerator and brake:

- lever extensions to blinkers, the gear shift, wipers
- a spinner knob, fork attachment or 'C' bar attachment to the steering wheel for steering
- extended lever, alternative grip, or alternate location for handbrake
- built-up key/push-button start or relocated ignition switch
- built-up handles, leather loops or metal ring attachments for controls on the dashboard
- alternative seatbelts for adequate restraints (harness, lapsash, additional chest strap—important for some quadriplegics, as retractable seat belts may be inappropriate)
- alternative handles for doors
- bench/bucket seat changes
- some emergency help indicator (CB radio or sign to request help if necessary)
- an electronic blinker control on the throttle or headrest

Modifications available in New South Wales

These can be carried out by many businesses, including:

John Anderson Auto Conversions
20 Taylors Road
DURAL NSW 2158
Tel.: (02) 651 3454

Paraquad Engineering
8 Hearne Street
MORTDALE NSW 2223
Tel.: (02) 534 3577

It is usually helpful to phone these businesses and discuss modifications and the cost.

Modifications available in other States and Territories

South Australia

Merv Jenkins
17 Towers Terrace
PLYMPTON SOUTH SA 5038
Tel.: (08) 297 2128

Owen Parker
6 Batley Crescent
PARA VISTA SA 5093
Tel.: (08) 264 1361

Portolde Hand Controls
Australian Technology Pty Ltd
36 Raglan Avenue
EDWARDSTOWN SA 5039
Tel.: (08) 297 1364

Victoria

Franks Engineering
84 Morell Street
GLENROY VIC 3046
Tel.: (03) 306 4399

Norden Transport Equipment
Bennett Street
DANDENONG VIC 3175

Mobile Tech
PO Box 466
NIDDYIC VIC 3042
Tel.: (03) 334 4522

Western Australia

Ben Ludlow
150 Railway Parade
BAYSWATER WA 6053

TL Engineering
300 Collier Road
BAYSWATER WA 6053

For information on car modifications in Queensland, Northern Territory, Tasmania and the Australian Capital Territory, contact the occupational therapy department at your local hospital.

■ Purchasing a car

The main form of government help to disabled people wishing to buy a car is sales tax exemption. This is administered by the Taxation Department:

Sales Tax (Motor Vehicle) Exemption Office
GPO Box 7047
SYDNEY NSW 2001
Tel.: (02) 236 7984

A disabled person is eligible for sales tax exemption on a new motor vehicle if he or she is able to produce evidence that the vehicle is necessary for employment. (Unfortunately, this concession is not available for attendance at a tertiary institution or rehabilitation centre.) Applications must be made through the Taxation Department.

The applications are then assessed together with information from the specialist or local doctor. Eligibility for the Department of Social Security's mobility allowance is revoked once sales tax exemption is granted. It is also possible to obtain sales tax exemption on motor vehicle parts through this scheme.

■ Driver's licences

A person who becomes disabled must notify the Road Traffic Authority and in some cases undergo an assessment in order to determine whether he or she is eligible for a driver's licence.

Driving assessments

You must obtain a medical form, available from the Road Traffic Authority, and have it completed by your treating doctor. This form can be lodged at your local Road Traffic Authority, or sent directly to:

The Medical Officer
Road Traffic Authority
ROSEBERY NSW 2018

The medical officer may:
- recommend that you are medically fit to drive a car with set conditions
- add to the conditions on the licence—for example, suggest appropriate car modifications
- request a physical examination and assess you on a driving simulator to see if you are capable of driving
- endorse your licence as a learners permit only. You will then be required to complete an on-road assessment. A written test may be requested

Disability driving assessments can be organised at any branch of the Road Traffic Authority. Once you have passed, a new licence will be issued stating the controls to be used.

Driver instruction in New South Wales

Driver instruction through private driving schools can be co-ordinated by the Commonwealth Rehabilitation Service or through the occupational therapy department at your local hospital.

Driver instruction in other States and Territories

South Australia
Department of Road Transport
60 Wakefield Street
ADELAIDE SA 5000
Tel.: (08) 226 7420

Victoria
Occupational Therapy Department
Austin Hospital
Studley Road
HEIDELBERG VIC 3084
Tel.: (03) 450 5105

Western Australia
Police Department of Western Australia
Cnr Wellington & Plain Streets
EAST PERTH WA 6004

In other States and Territories, the occupational therapist at the spinal injuries unit will have details.

'Disabled' signs

It is not necessary to display these, but some people prefer to do so or at least carry one in case they may need it at some time in an emergency. The signs are available from the Paraplegic and Quadriplegic Association of New South Wales.

■ Disabled parking authority in New South Wales

This authority, administered by the Road Traffic Authority, allows a person to park for an extended period in a time-limited parking zone (without having to pay, if it is a metered area). This does not apply to 'No stopping/No parking' areas. Application forms are available at local Road Traffic Authority offices. Forms need to be completed by the applicant and his or her doctor.

Disabled parking authority in other States and Territories

Queensland
Department of Transport
230 Brunswick Street
FORTITUDE VALLEY QLD 4006

South Australia
Motor Registration
60 Wakefield Street
ADELAIDE SA 5000
Tel.: (08) 226 7400

Victoria
Contact your local council for further information.

Western Australia
ACROD
189 Royal Street
EAST PERTH WA 6004

Residents of Tasmania, the Australian Capital Territory and Northern Territory should contact the social work departments at their local hospitals.

Taxi Transport Subsidy Scheme in New South Wales

This is a scheme to provide low-cost taxi transport for disabled persons, especially those in wheelchairs. It is administered by:

> The Department of Transport
> GPO Box 1620
> SYDNEY NSW 2001
> Tel.: (02) 963 0325

The scheme runs a number of wheelchair-accessible taxis that operate on a 24-hour-day, seven-day-week basis. It is especially designed to help those people who are permanently unable to use buses, ferries and trains.

The scheme operates in the centres of Sydney, Newcastle and Wollongong, and in major country towns of New South Wales. People accepted into this scheme are provided with an identity card and a specially encoded voucher that entitles them to use the taxi and pay only half fare.

Application should be made to the Department of Transport, which asks for personal details and a doctor's statement of disability.

Taxi transport subsidies in other States and Territories

Queensland

> Department of Transport
> 230 Brunswick Street
> FORTITUDE VALLEY QLD 4006

South Australia

> Transport Subsidy Scheme
> Office of Transport Policy and Planning
> GPO Box 1599
> ADELAIDE SA 5001

Victoria

> Victoria Roads
> Multi Purpose Taxi Program
> Tel.: (03) 345 4105

Western Australia

> Department of Transport (WA)
> 136 Stirling Highway
> NEDLANDS WA 6009

Residents of Tasmania, the Australian Capital Territory and Northern Territory should contact the social work department of their local hospitals.

Air travel

Most airlines are geared for carrying disabled passengers. Special considerations do, however, need to be kept in mind. The following is a list of steps needed for travel with Qantas. (Most airlines have a similar system.)

■ Travelling overseas with Qantas

These are the steps you should take (ring Qantas Enquiries and Reservations on (02) 957 0111):

- Decide where and when you want to travel.
- Book your trip as usual through a travel agent.
- Obtain a 'Fitness to Travel' form from Qantas or your travel agent. This provides the airline with medical information about your disability. Fill it out and return it to Qantas as soon as possible— no later than four days before you are due to leave. The Qantas medical department uses the 'Fitness to Travel' form as a guide to any special arrangements that the airline may need to make for your trip.

Note that wheelchairs are not charged as excess luggage, and can also be provided. You can make pre-seating arrangements.

■ Travel on domestic airlines

Ansett

> Domestic reservations:
> Tel.: (02) 268 1111

Ansett has established the ANSACARE system, to simplify flight arrangements for disabled people. Personal details and special requirements are stored on computer, within the reservation system.

Applicants are issued with an ANSACARE card. When booking a flight, quote your personal ANSACARE number, thus alerting Ansett of your special needs and eliminating the need to obtain medical clearance for each trip.

Australian Airlines

> Domestic reservations:
> Tel.: (02) 693 3333

On application, you can have details of your disability recorded on computer.

For both domestic airlines, application forms can be obtained by contacting your closest airline office. Wheelchairs are not charged as excess luggage.

■ At the airport

Take your own wheelchair. When you arrive at the airport this will need to be replaced by an airport chair, designed to fit into the plane. Your own chair will be stored as part of your luggage in the hold.

You will board the plane either through the air bridge or through a special lift.

You will find that most airlines now have an understanding of the special seating and toilet requirements of disabled people.

CHAPTER 15

Recreation

Rehabilitation aims at helping people to increase their level of independence and sense of self-worth. Returning to work is often seen as the ultimate achievement in the rehabilitation process. However, while work itself has many benefits, it is equally important to find value and enjoyment in your leisure time, especially if your disability makes it difficult for you to obtain employment.

Having too much leisure time and no interests is an ingredient for boredom and depression. It reinforces the feelings of failure and helplessness. On the other hand, being interested and involved in an activity helps you to forget your problems, and may leave you relaxed and revitalised.

The challenge is to find which recreational activities give you pleasure and fulfilment. Some activities may need no changes at all from their original form, while others may appear impossible to do. If you are motivated and use a little imagination, you will be surprised at how many activities can be adapted or modified. You might consider the following.

Sports associations

■ New South Wales

There are a number of sporting activities available to the spinal-injured person. Not only is sport a great way to exercise, but it is also a good way to meet new people and make friends. Basketball, table tennis, track and field, archery and tennis are all sports that are readily available to wheelchair sportspersons.

The list of sporting groups and associations is long, and can be found in the *Yellow Pages*. If you would like more information about sports, it would be advisable to contact:

NSW Wheelchair Sports Association
600 Victoria Road
RYDE NSW 2112
Tel.: (02) 809 5260

This club conducts regular competitions, meetings and training days in many, varied sports, for all standards—from beginner to international competition level.

The club now has its own premises:

The Sports Stadium
Mount Street
MT DRUITT NSW 2770,

where regular basketball competitions are conducted for players of all standards on Thursday nights. There is also a magazine sent regularly to members, called the *Pushers Post*, which contains details of many different activities planned by the club.

Membership costs $15.00.

The Association also co-ordinates the Qantas Oz-Day 10 km race, which is an international wheelchair road race held every Australia Day in Sydney, attracting competitors from all over Australia and around the world.

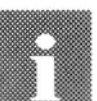 ## Other States and Territories

Queensland

The Sporting Wheelies and Disabled Sport and
Recreation Association of Queensland
24 Ross Street
NEWSTEAD QLD 4006

South Australia

Wheelchair Sports Association
Hampstead Centre
Folland Avenue
NORTHFIELD SA 5085

Recreation Association for People with Disabilities
c/- Walkerville YMCA
39 Smith Street
WALKERVILLE SA 5081
Tel.: (08) 344 3811

Victoria

Wheelchair Sports Victoria
Tel.: (03) 329 5088

Western Australia

WA Wheelchair Sports Association
Sussex Street
VICTORIA PARK WA 6100

Residents in Tasmania, Northern Territory and the Australian Capital Territory should contact the occupational therapy departments at their local hospitals, or telephone NICAN (see below).

Sports magazines

Sports n' Spoke is a magazine exclusively dealing with wheelchair sports and recreation. It has up-to-date information on the latest recreational opportunities, plus complete coverage of competitive wheelchair sports. It presents features on active disabled people and interesting articles on new equipment, conditioning and fitness. Subscriptions may be sent to:

Paralysed Veterans of America
Paraplegic News/Sports n' Spoke
5201N 19th Avenue
Suite 111
PHOENIX ARIZONA 85015 USA

Accessible Arts Network

NSW Writers Centre
Rozelle Hospital
Balmain Road
PO Box 1022
ROZELLE NSW 2029
Tel.: (02) 555 1022

This is a community arts project involving people with disabilities, artists and the community. It aims to provide workshops and information on creative arts for individuals and community groups. Workshop topics include drama, dance, music, mime, puppetry, computer graphics, computer music, screen printing, visual arts, craft, sculptural landscaping and ceramics.

In this way, Network hopes to act as a springboard from which people can develop ideas and projects and the confidence to pursue creative activities themselves.

Reading Library Service

Reading is one activity that most people enjoy. A continuous and cheap source of supply of reading material is available at your local library. A number of libraries throughout New South Wales also have services for assisting disabled people.

Here are examples of these services.

■ Talking books

These are cassette tapes of books. Anyone may borrow them.

■ Home/hospital/community services

Librarians may arrange for helpers to deliver books to disabled people at home or in hospital. Not all libraries have these services, but if you would like to use them, or get such a service established, why not contact the chief librarian at your local library? (Libraries are run by local municipal councils, and are listed in the 'Local Government' section of the *White Pages*.)

Gardening and horticulture

Gardening can be creative and relaxing. There is growing interest by disabled people in this recreational activity, with the opportunity to develop skills through the following centres and courses.

■ Banksia Centre

Australian Botanic Gardens
Black Mountain
PO Box 158
CANBERRA ACT 2601

This centre has been set up to teach disabled people the art of gardening. It also helps people to modify their gardens and select appropriate tools.

■ Hydroponics course

The Australian Quadriplegic Association
LITTLE BAY NSW 2036
Tel.: (02) 661 8855

AQA offers a six month part-time course, created by and for people with disabilities, on hydroponic gardening (growing plants without soil).

Outdoor recreation

The Australian bush is a very special place, and spending time in it can be really relaxing. The New South Wales National Parks and Wildlife Service has produced a booklet, 'Outdoor Access for Everyone', which lists over 190 places within the New South Wales National Park system that are wheelchair-accessible. Bush trails, camping sites, waterfalls, lookouts, picnic areas, historic buildings and museums are described, with details of their facilities and accessibility. Copies of the booklet can be obtained from:

The New South Wales National Parks and Wildlife
  Service
43 Bridge Street
HURSTVILLE NSW 2220
Tel.: (02) 585 6444

■ Outward Bound Australia

This is an adventure recreation association that has developed courses for people with disabilities. Details of courses, which include exploration of the bush through camping, canoeing and a variety of other activities, can be obtained from:

Outward Bound Australia
630 George Street
SYDNEY NSW 2001
Tel.: (02) 261 2200

Holidays

Holidays are a great way to relax and feel refreshed. Increasingly, as people are becoming aware of the needs of the disabled person, more provision is being made by the travel industry for accommodating these needs.

Several accommodation books and pamphlets are available. These include:

* *Accommodation for the Disabled Traveller in Australia*, compiled by the Department of Industry and Commerce, and available from the Tourism Division in Canberra of this department
* *Accommodation Directory*, compiled by the NRMA. Wheelchair-accessible accommodation is listed. This information is available through the NRMA's branch offices

Booklets have been published for all capital cities in Australia, and give details of accessible buildings, shops etc. in each city. They are available through bookshops in all States.

■ Travel agents

There are two travel agents in Sydney that specialise in travel for the disabled both overseas and in Australia:

Crossroads Travel
44 Margaret Street
SYDNEY NSW 2000
Tel.: (02) 262 1811

Cumalong Tours
PO Box 224
NORTHBRIDGE NSW 2063
Tel.: (02) 958 8379

■ Travel companies

Most travel organisations are starting to make provision for disabled people. Contact them to make inquiries.

Directories

For a more comprehensive listing of recreation choices, use the *Directory of Recreation Resources for People with Disabilities*, produced by the New South Wales government. It includes details on art, crafts, sports, holidays, camps and transport. The directory is available from:

The Department of Sport and Recreation
PO Box 1032
BURWOOD NORTH NSW 2134
Tel.: (02) 747 2655

NICAN

Another way of finding out information about leisure and recreation activities is through NICAN (the National Information Communication Awareness Network). The NICAN Database is an on-line directory providing information about leisure activities for people with disabilities. Requests for information can be made through your local library (if it is linked to the directory), or by writing to:

NICAN Information Centre
Freepost 284
CANBERRA ACT 2601
Tel. (reverse charges): (06) 285 3713

CHAPTER 16

Discrimination—knowing your rights

People who discriminate against others usually do so out of ignorance, or because they are uncomfortable with other people being different from themselves. That difference may be racial, sexual, religious, intellectual or physical. Though attitudes *are* changing, there may still be times when you feel you have been treated unfairly (i.e. you are discriminated against) simply because you have a spinal injury and perhaps use a wheelchair or walking aids.

Having a spinal injury does not mean that your rights have changed. To ensure that people with disabilities are not discriminated against, the New South Wales government has introduced anti-discrimination laws. The following information about these laws in New South Wales is provided by the New South Wales Anti-Discrimination Board, which is responsible for their administration.

Is discrimination against people with physical disabilities against the law?

Yes, it is. In New South Wales it is generally against the law for people either to treat you unfairly or to harass you because you have a physical disability or a physical illness that has affected your body's structure or functioning.

It is against the law for people to do this:

- for most types of employment—when you apply for a job, at any time during your employment, or when you are already in a job
- when you try to get most types of goods and services—for example, from shops, pubs and entertainment places, banks, lawyers, government departments, doctors or hospitals
- when you rent, or try to rent, accommodation—for example, a unit, house or commercial premises, or a hotel or motel room
- when you apply to get into, or are already studying in, any State education institution—a university, college, TAFE or State school
- when you try to enter or join a registered club, or when you visit one (a registered club includes any club that sells alcohol or has gambling machines)

What are my rights?

■ Employment

You have the right:

- to compete for jobs and promotions on the same terms as everyone else—that is, in relation to your ability to do the job, your qualifications and your experience. For example, questions on application forms and at interviews must be about your ability to do the particular job, not about your disability. Employers can only rely on medical information that is directly relevant to your ability to carry out the duties of the particular job
- to expect your employer to make any 'reasonable' adjustments to the work environment that are necessary to accommodate your disability
- not to be harassed about your disability when you apply for a job, when you are at work, or when you leave a job

■ Obtaining goods and services

You have the right:

- generally to be able to get goods and services in the same way as people who do not have a disability. For example, providers must not refuse you service just because you are in a wheelchair—unless it is physically impossible to give you access to the place where the service is located. If your disability means that you can't drive, service providers who need identification from you must not insist that only a driving licence will do

- not to be harassed about your disability when you are obtaining goods or services

■ Renting accommodation

You have the right:

- generally to rent any accommodation, on the same terms as anyone else. People can only refuse you accommodation because of your disability if it is impossible for them to provide you with access to the accommodation, or if you would be at risk of injury if you used it
- not to be harassed because of your disability by a real-estate agent or owner when you apply to rent or are renting accommodation

■ State education

You have the right:

- generally to study at any State educational institution in the same way as any other student. Institutions can only refuse to enrol you because of your disability if you need either special services or adjustments made to the building that they can not 'reasonably' provide.

  Institutions must make 'reasonable' adjustments to allow you to sit for tests and examinations, and it is 'reasonable' for them to make sure that your classes are in rooms that are both accessible to you and near enough to each other to allow you to get to each class
- not to be harassed because of your disability when you apply to study at, or are studying at, any State educational institution

■ Registered clubs

You have the right:

- generally to join, enter or get services in registered clubs on the same terms as everyone else. Clubs can only refuse you membership or entry if you need special facilities that they cannot 'reasonably' provide. If you want to dance on the dance floor in a wheelchair, this should generally be allowed—unless it is unsafe
- not to be harassed because of your disability when you try to enter or join, or are inside, any registered club

ℹ What can I do if I am treated unfairly or harassed because of my disability?

If this happens to you, and you cannot sort it out yourself, please phone, write to or visit the Anti-Discrimination Board. The Board has the legal power to investigate your complaint, and, if what has happened to you is against the law, to conciliate it—that is, to help you and the person or the organisation you're complaining about to reach a private settlement that you both agree on.

The settlement will depend on the circumstances of your case. It could be financial compensation, it could be that you are considered for a job, it could be that an education program is run to ensure that people with disabilities are not discriminated against by that organisation in future, and so on.

The Board's officers treat all complaints confidentially, and its services are free. The Board will not contact the organisation or person you are complaining about unless you are sure that is what you want it to do. And it is against the law for anyone to hassle or 'victimise' you because you have complained to the Anti-Discrimination Board.

Most complaints are conciliated. If yours is not, you may go to the Equal Opportunity Tribunal—a court that provides a legal judgment that must be followed. However, very, very few cases need to go to court.

For more information, or to make a complaint, contact:

The Anti-Discrimination Board of New South Wales (open weekdays 9 a.m. to 5 p.m.)

Level 4
181 Lawson Street
REDFERN NSW 2016
Tel.: (02) 318 5400
Fax: (02) 310 2235

TTY (telephone typewriter for deaf or hearing impaired persons):
Tel.: (02) 310 2376

The Redfern office is wheelchair-accessible. There is parking nearby for people with disabilities—phone for details.

84 Crown Street
WOLLONGONG NSW 2500
Tel.: (042) 26 8190
Fax: (042) 26 1190

The Wollongong office is wheelchair-accessible. Phone if parking required, as this can be arranged.

79 Hunter Street
NEWCASTLE NSW 2300
Tel.: (049) 26 4300
Fax: (049) 26 1376

Access to the Newcastle office is by one small step on entry to the building.

ℹ The Disability Complaints Service

Another way of making a complaint if you believe your rights have been infringed is through the Disability Complaints Service:

Suite 5
Level 8
Strathfield Plaza
The Boulevarde
STRATHFIELD NSW 2135
Tel.: (008) 42 4007 or (02) 746 3230

TTY—typewriter telephone number:

(02) 764 3485

Fax: (02) 746 3262

The Disability Complaints Service is sponsored by Disabled Persons International (New South Wales) Inc. and is an independent, free advocacy and information service for people with disabilities or those acting on their behalf. You can make a complaint about any service you have received or any situation where you think your rights have not been recognised or respected.

If it is more appropriate that the complaint be handled by an existing service (such as the Anti-Discrimination Board), the Disability Complaints Service will refer you to that service for advice. The Disability Complaints Service will also provide the support you need to use that service and will monitor the progress of your complaint.

This organisation keeps all information about complaints confidential, and no information can be released without the permission of the person making the complaint.

Commonwealth government laws

In the near future, the Commonwealth government will consider introducing national legislation that will prohibit discrimination against people with disabilities. Though anti-discrimination laws already exist in New South Wales, Victoria, South Australia and Western Australia, people with disabilities in Queensland, Tasmania, the Northern Territory and the Australian Capital Territory have no such protection.

The proposed legislation would not invalidate existing State laws, but would cover those areas of discrimination, such as access to public transport, for which there are as yet no provisions.

For further information on the proposed legislation, contact your local Federal Member of Parliament.

Anti-discrimination organisations in States and Territories other than New South Wales

South Australia

Disability Complaints Service
62A Henly Beach Road
MILE END SA 5031
Tel.: (08) 234 5699

Victoria

Equal Opportunities Commission
Tel.: (03) 602 3085

Western Australia

Equal Opportunities Commission
5 Mill Street
PERTH WA 6000

Index